D1448046

Coping with

Coping with Aging Series

Series Editors
John C. Rosenbek, Ph.D.
Chief, Speech Pathology and Audiology Services
William S. Middleton Memorial Hospital
Madison, Wisconsin

Medical Editor
Molly Carnes, M.D.
Department of Medicine and Institute on Aging
University of Wisconsin
Madison, Wisconsin

Associate Director for Clinical Services
Geriatric Research, Education and Clinical Center
William S. Middleton Memorial Hospital
Madison, Wisconsin

Published in Cooperation with
the National Council of Senior Citizens

Published by Singular Publishing Group, Inc.
4284 41st Street
San Diego, California 92105-1197

©1994 by Singular Publishing Group, Inc.

Illustrations by Loralee A. McAuliffe

Typeset in 11/14 Times by So Cal Graphics
Printed in the United States of America by BookCrafters

Library of Congress Cataloging-in-Publication Data

Mahoney, Jane.
    Coping with impaired mobility/ Jane Mahoney, Reenie Euhardy.
      p.   cm. — (Coping with aging series)
    Includes bibliographical references and index.
    ISBN 1-879105-65-9
    1. Musculoskeletal diseases in old age. 2. Movement disorders.
  3. Physical therapy for the aged. I. Euhardy, Reenie. II. Title
  III. Series
RC925.53.M34   1994
618.97'67—dc20   93-40443
                                         CIP

Coping with Impaired Mobility

Jane Mahoney M.D.
Geriatrician

Reenie Euhardy P.T.
Physical Therapist
Geriatric Clinical Specialist

SINGULAR PUBLISHING GROUP, INC.
SAN DIEGO, CALIFORNIA

❖ Table of Contents

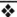

❖ Foreword

The books in the *Coping with Aging Series* are written for men and women coping with the challenges of aging, and for their families and other caregivers. The authors are all experienced practitioners: doctors, nurses, social workers, psychologists, pharmacists, nutritionists, audiologists, physical and occupational therapists, and speech-language pathologists.

The topics of individual volumes are as varied as are the challenges that aging may bring. These include: hearing loss, low vision, depression, sexual dysfunction, immobility, intellectual impairment, language impairment, speech impairment, swallowing impairment, death and dying, bowel and bladder incontinence, stress of caregiving, giving up independence, medications, and stroke. The volumes themselves, however, share common features. Foremost, they are practical, jargon-free, and responsible. Each contains professionally valid information translated into language people who are not health care providers can understand. Each contains useful advice and sections to help readers decide how they are doing and whether they need to do more, do less, or do something different. Each provides evidence that no single person need cope alone.

None of the volumes can substitute for appropriate professional health care. However, when combined with the care, instruction, and counseling that health care providers supply, they make coping with aging easier. America is greying at the same time its treasury is inadequate to meet its population's needs. Thus the *Coping with Aging Series* offers help for people who need and want to help themselves.

This book, *Coping with Impaired Mobility*, is written by two professionals in geriatrics. Dr. Mahoney is a geriatrician with particular experience in treating older adults with mobility problems. Reenie Euhardy is a physical therapist and a certified clinical specialist in geriatrics. If you or someone you know has a problem with mobility, this book will be helpful. You will find out what can be done to improve the ability to move around and how to cope if moving is difficult or impossible. You will discover how to reduce the risk of falls and what to do if a fall does occur. You will find lists of specific stretching, strengthening, and balance training exercises. You will learn about medical conditions such as arthritis, osteoporosis, and diabetes that can have an impact on mobility. The language is straightforward and clear. The lesson is that specific things can be done to prevent immobility, reduce its severity when it does occur, and cope with the restrictions that cannot be prevented.

John C. Rosenbek, Ph.D.
Series Editor

Molly Carnes, M.D.
Medical Editor

❖ Preface

Mobility means different things to different people. For some people it means being able to walk a mile a day. For others, mobility means being able to go to church or to the store; for still others it means simply being able to get around inside the house. Whatever *your* level of mobility, this book is concerned with helping you remain as mobile and independent as you possibly can.

The first six chapters of this book cover aspects of mobility which apply to all older people, whether healthy or frail. These chapters discuss the role of balance, strength, posture, and flexibility in keeping you mobile and active. Chapters 2 through 5 include exercises to help you improve in each of these areas of mobility, and Chapter 6 gives conditioning activities to help you maintain or increase your overall level of fitness. For most of the exercises and activities, several variations are described so that the intensity of each workout can be adapted to suit your needs.

Several chapters are devoted to specific problems that can affect your mobility. The common problems of dizziness and unsteadiness, arthritis, and osteoporosis are examined in detail in Chapters 7, 8, and 9. Hints are given on how best to cope with these conditions, when you can self-treat, and when you should seek medical advice. Chapter 10 discusses how a number of other medical conditions, as well as many medications, can limit your mobility. Each chapter includes practical suggestions on ways to enhance your activity level.

Chapters 11 and 12 discuss in detail how important healthy feet and good footwear are for your mobility. Common foot disorders which can make walking painful or difficult are described, as are the types of shoes that are indicated for various foot problems. Tips are included on what to look for when purchasing new shoes and how to determine if new shoes fit you correctly.

Many people use canes or other types of ambulation aids to enhance their mobility. Chapter 13 describes the many types of canes and walkers that are available and the different styles of wheelchairs and electric scooters you can choose from. No walking aid is necessarily better than another. The pros and cons of each device are reviewed.

The final chapter deals with falls, which are all too common a problem for older adults. Why falling is such a concern for older people and the effect falls often have on mobility are explained. There are many things that you can do to reduce the risk of falling. By simply following the suggestions in Chapter 14 on home safety and paying attention to the tips given in previous chapters about maintaining your mobility, you can reduce the risk of falling.

The information included in the chapters is presented in an upbeat and encouraging style. The material is useful and easy to understand, and medical jargon has been eliminated. Throughout the book, coping with immobility is discussed in a practical manner with down-to-earth advice that will allow you to remain as active as possible.

❖ Acknowledgments

The authors would like to acknowledge Neil Binkley, M.D., Alan J. Kalker, D.P.M., and Brian Mink, C.O., for their review of parts of the manuscript. The authors also would like to give a special thank you to their husbands and sons for all their patience and support.

Chapter 1

Balance and Strength

What Is Balance?

Balance is what you do to keep yourself upright with your
weight over your center of gravity. Without a sense of balance you would not be able to walk or even sit in an
upright position. Although a sense of balance for most
people is automatic, something you do without thinking,
it actually is a very complex activity. You can think of balance as being composed of two types of actions. The first
type of action is what you do to keep from falling over
when you are standing still. This is called "static balance."
The second type is what you do to keep yourself balanced
when you are moving. This is called "dynamic balance."

What Does Balance Consist Of?

You can think of balance as a three-part mechanism. First,
your senses collect input from your surroundings and your
body; second, your brain processes that input; and finally, your
muscles produce the output needed to keep you from falling.

How Your Senses Affect Balance

Every time you adjust your balance, you are doing it in
response to input from your senses. For example, you see
that the sidewalk is uneven and feel that it is icy. You
depend on your senses to obtain this information. The
senses that are most important for balance are vision,
touch, joint position sense, and inner ear function. This
section discusses how these senses change with age, and

how these changes may affect your balance. It also gives you helpful hints for getting the most information you can from your senses.

Vision

Vision is an important part of balance. Poor vision will make it harder for you to maintain your balance. With limited eyesight you may be afraid of falling, even to the point of cutting back on your activities.

The best thing you can do to make sure you are not developing a vision problem is to get regular eye check-ups. Not all vision problems are simply the result of aging, and vision loss often is curable. With regular eye examinations treatable vision problems can be found early *before* they affect your mobility. Chapter 10 discusses some of the common, treatable eye diseases that can interfere with your vision.

Certain eyesight changes are a normal part of aging and are not treatable. These are discussed under the headings of glare, light and dark accommodation, peripheral vision, and seeing close objects.

Glare

The pupil adjusts the amount of light entering the eye. To see properly, the pupils need to constrict when the light is bright. With age, the pupils constrict more slowly. Therefore, as you age it becomes harder to adjust to bright light. This means that glare becomes more bothersome and will seem even brighter to you than it did when you were young. Glossy surfaces such as waxed linoleum or wood floors can increase glare and make it harder to see where you are walking. At night, glare may be even more of a problem because artificial lighting can be especially harsh.

What You Can Do. If glare bothers you, or if you already have trouble with eyesight or balance, you should not have a high gloss shine or wax on your floors at home, because this increases glare. When you are walking on surfaces where there is a lot of glare, pay close attention to your walking. If you concentrate closely on your walking and balance, you will be much less likely to trip, even if conditions are not optimal for your vision.

Light and Dark Accommodation

Your pupil not only takes longer to adjust to bright lights, it also takes longer to dilate as the eye adjusts to the dark when you are older. As you go from a lighted to a dark room it may become much more difficult for you to see. This is especially true at night when there are different intensities of light in different rooms. During the day it can be a problem if you leave a bright sunlit kitchen and go downstairs into a dark basement.

What You Can Do. The most important thing you can do is to make sure you have good lighting in and around your home so that you will be able to see as well as possible. You should never walk or move around in the dark. If you have to go into areas where lighting is dim, give your eyes plenty of time to adjust before you start moving around. Also, remember that if the lighting is dim, you will need to pay extra attention to where you are walking to avoid tripping over obstacles you may not readily see.

Peripheral Vision

Peripheral vision decreases somewhat with normal aging. A loss of peripheral vision may affect your ability to see things "out of the corner of your eye." It is easy to lose your balance and fall if you do not notice obstacles in your path. For instance, you may be less likely to notice where the corner of the bed is if you are looking straight ahead as you walk around the bed to make it.

What You Can Do. To compensate for a loss in peripheral vision you need to take more care to watch your feet when you walk. Glance to the sides frequently while walking to be sure you see objects around you. Turning your head slightly from side to side as you scan your surroundings will help make up for limited peripheral vision.

Seeing Close Objects

Everyone has more trouble seeing objects close to them as they age. This is farsightedness, also known as the "my arms are too short disease." This phrase refers to having to hold printed materials at arm's length to read them. As farsightedness progresses, your arms are not long enough to hold things far enough away so you can read them! Treatment for this universal condition is the use of glasses, bifocals, contact lenses, or magnifying lenses.

Being farsighted will not cause you any difficulty seeing the ground in front of you, because seeing objects at the distance of your feet is not affected. However, wearing glasses that correct for farsightedness can affect your mobility. Glasses that correct farsightedness make objects appear closer than they are. Reading glasses may distort the way you see the floor and make you prone to tripping.

Bifocals can create the same type of problem, especially on stairs. When walking down stairs, there is a natural tendency to look through the bottom of the bifocals. Because this part of the lens magnifies objects, it will make stair steps look larger and closer to you than they really are. It is easy to misjudge the height of steps and fall if you are not extra cautious.

What You Can Do. Wearing your reading glasses for activities other than reading and close work is not a good idea. If you are wearing bifocals when you are going down stairs, you will need to make a conscious effort to look through the *top* not the bottom half of your bifocals. To do this, you will need to bend your head down a little more than you normally would. If you are looking out of the top of your bifocals, but continue to have a problem on stairs, instead of wearing bifocals you may need to get two pairs of glasses. One pair of glasses can be used for reading and a different pair can be used for walking and doing other activities that require distant vision.

Sense of Touch

Nerves pick up information from the skin in your feet and carry this information to the brain. These nerves give you your sense of touch so that you can feel the ground you are walking on. If you have a problem with these nerves, you may have difficulty walking. Some older adults may have a slight decrease in their sense of touch as they age. Certain diseases also can cause a loss of the sense of touch.

Testing Your Sense of Touch

One way to test the sense of touch in your feet is to take a wisp of cotton and lightly touch your feet and then your hand. Some people, when they get older, will not feel a light touch as well on their foot as they do on their hand.

Sometimes a decrease in the sensitivity of the nerves is due to a significant medical problem instead. This type of nerve loss tends to be more severe. To test for this, if you had trouble feeling the wisp of cotton, try a broom bristle. If you have trouble feeling the touch of a broom bristle on your foot, you should consult your doctor, because you may have an underlying medical condition. Some of the medical problems that can cause nerve damage are discussed in Chapter 7.

What You Can Do. Because your sense of touch may become less sharp as you age, it is very important to compensate for this by paying more attention to the surface you are walking on. Always watch where you are stepping, particularly if the ground is uneven or slippery. You also may need to slow down your movements, especially on rough surfaces, because you will not detect subtle irregularities on the ground and can easily stumble and lose your balance.

Another way to compensate if your sense of touch becomes less sharp is to make sure that areas where you walk are as safe as possible. In your home, pick up loose throw rugs and put a nonskid bath mat in the tub. Chapter 14 includes a home safety checklist to help you decrease your risk of falling by eliminating hazards in your home.

Joint Position Sense

Nerves also help you to know how your body is positioned. For example, when you close your eyes, nerves in your joints tell you if your arm is hanging down by your side or raised out in front of you. About one third of elderly people have some abnormality of position sense. They may not even be aware of it, but when specifically tested by a physician or therapist, they will have a problem detecting subtle changes in body position. Problems with position sense are not usually a part of normal aging, but they frequently are the result of various diseases that occur in older people. Regardless of the cause, difficulty with position sense will affect your ability to balance, especially with your eyes closed.

Testing Your Joint Position Sense

It is difficult for you to evaluate your own joint position sense. You may have a loss of joint position sense in some joints but not others. A physician can determine which joints, if any, you have a problem with.

What You Can Do. If you have a problem with joint position sense, you subconsciously will start to rely more on other senses, particularly vision, to help you maintain your balance. The best way to compensate for a loss of joint position sense is to make sure the lighting around you is good and to be careful and attentive when you walk or move around. Use your eyes to help tell you specifically where your feet are. For example, are you raising your foot high enough to clear an uneven crack in the sidewalk or to step over a door threshold?

Inner Ear

The inner ear contains special sensors that tell your brain when and how your head is moving. These sensors are called hair cells. When you tilt your head back and look up at the ceiling, hair cells detect this head movement and relay this information to your brain. These sensors are very important in helping you keep your balance as you turn or move your head.

As you age your inner ear loses some of its function and does not detect head motion as well as it used to. The total number of hair cells decreases and each hair cell must feel more movement before it can detect a change. For most people these changes in the function of the inner ear with aging are so small that they are insignificant. This is because you can also rely on your eyesight, and on your senses of touch and joint position, to help you keep your balance. You may notice a problem only when it is dark and you can't rely on your eyesight to help you balance.

Many older people, however, also have problems with vision or have lost some of their sense of touch and joint position sense. If you have problems with these other senses, you may find your balance affected because you cannot compensate as well for your loss of inner ear function.

Testing Your Inner Ear Function

You can check for some types of inner ear problems by a simple test. While sitting, bend your head back and look up at the ceiling. Then turn your head to the side while you continue to look at the ceiling with your head back. If these movements give you the feeling that you are moving, spinning, or losing your balance, or that the room is spinning or moving, you may have a significant problem with your inner ear.

CAUTION: Do not do this test if you have severe neck arthritis or a problem with fainting. Bending your head back can aggravate arthritis or precipitate a black-out spell.

What You Can Do

One way to compensate for a loss of inner ear function is to be extra cautious of your balance when you are moving your head. Be aware that when you bend your head to look up or down, you are more likely to become unsteady. Try not to make quick head movements when you are walking because this can throw you off balance. Also, hold onto something for support before you attempt to tilt your head back to look up at things over your head.

Summary

A number of normal age–related changes in your vision, touch, and inner ear function can affect your balance. You can improve your balance, however, simply by being aware of your movements and taking extra care to avoid falling as you walk and move around. Being extra careful is especially important when there is poor lighting or the environment is hazardous, such as when the sidewalk is wet and slippery.

You also can do exercises and participate in activities to improve your balance. Chapter 2 describes some specific exercises and activities you can do to improve your sense of balance.

How Your Brain Affects Balance

The brain takes all the information it receives from your eyes, your feet, your joints, and your inner ear and puts it all together. It does this every second, whether you are standing still or moving. Without the brain's work of organizing all this information, you would fall over when you stand in one position, and you would be unable to move without losing your balance. Whenever you walk, climb stairs, or do any kind of movement your brain is processing sensory input to ensure you keep your balance.

Reaction Time

The time it takes for the brain to process information increases as you get older, so it takes longer for the brain to respond to input from your senses. This means it takes you more time to react to a perceived danger. For example, in the winter when there is ice on the sidewalk, it will take you longer to perceive the ice and process this information. Therefore, it will take you longer to slow your walking pace in response.

Many medications also slow reaction time. If you have fallen, or have trouble with your balance, it may be related to some of the medications you are taking. Medications that can affect your balance are discussed in Chapter 10.

What You Can Do

Because your reaction time slows down when you get older, you will need to slow down your movements and take smaller steps, particularly when you are walking on uneven or slippery surfaces or in an unfamiliar environment. If you are taking medications, you should check with your doctor to see if they may be affecting your balance.

Balance exercises can help improve your movements. As you practice movements over and over again, you become more skilled in doing them and can do them more quickly. Specific balance exercises and activities are described in detail in Chapter 2.

How Your Muscles Affect Balance

The final part of balance is what your muscles do to keep you from falling. The effectiveness of your muscles in maintaining your balance is related to how strong they are. Muscle strength tends to decline as people get older. This decline in strength is due primarily to the fact that, as muscles age, they cannot generate force as effectively.

At the same time, as you get older the amount of muscle you have decreases. Even if your weight does not change, as you grow older, your body composition changes. The proportion of your body that is muscle decreases and the proportion that is fat increases.

Studies have shown that strength in the leg muscles, especially those that move the ankle, stays about the same until age 60 and then slowly decreases. By the time people reach their nineties, their muscle strength is decreased to half of what it was in their twenties. As your muscle strength declines, it affects both your balance and mobility. For example, if you start to lose your balance and fall backwards, your lower leg muscles help to pull you forward. Many older adults do not have the lower leg strength they need to prevent a backward fall.

If your thigh muscles are weak, you may find it very difficult to get up out of a chair. With weak thighs, in addition to feeling unsteady, you may be prone to losing your balance when you try to stand up from a chair or bed. Climbing stairs requires both thigh and buttock strength. Trying to go up stairs or up a curb may become unsafe if these muscles get too weak.

Testing Your Muscle Strength

You can test your leg muscle strength yourself by a couple of simple maneuvers. See if you can stand up from sitting in a chair without using your arms. If you need to use your arms for support, you probably have some thigh muscle weakness and you could benefit from thigh strengthening exercises. Next try to rise on your tiptoes.

You should be able to do this five times in a row. If you cannot do it five times, you could benefit from exercises to strengthen your calf muscles.

What You Can Do

By following a strengthening exercise program, the normal muscle loss that occurs with age can be greatly reduced. Weight lifting to increase your strength can be done even if you are in your nineties! Regardless of your age, if you start a weight training program, both muscle size and strength can be increased. Chapter 3 gives you detailed strengthening exercises designed for leg muscles and tells you how to go about starting a training program.

Summary

Good balance is essential to remaining active and mobile. Balance includes input from your senses, processing of those inputs by your brain, and finally the output from your muscles in response to the signals from your brain. All of these components of balance are affected by age. Although your balance tends to worsen as you get older, there are things you can do to decrease the risk of losing your balance and falling. Exercises and activities to improve your balance are described in the next chapter.

Chapter 2

Balance Exercises

If your mobility is impaired and you have problems with unsteadiness, balance exercises may help you. By improving your coordination and sense of balance, these exercises may allow you to move toward a more active lifestyle.

Why Will Balance Exercises Help?

Balance exercises are designed to improve the way your brain processes the information it gets from your senses. When you do balance exercises, your brain is practicing how to coordinate and organize all the information it has gotten from your eyes, feet, and joints. Your brain also is coordinating the messages it sends out to your muscles so that they work in a smooth fashion to keep you from falling.

Think of how dancers practice the same balance exercises over and over to learn how to maintain a difficult pose. The first time dancers try to stand on tiptoe, they cannot keep their balance. But when they practice the same movement over and over, they develop the skill to balance while rising up on their toes. In just the same way, if you are having trouble with your balance, you can work on movements you find difficult. By practicing these movements over and over, you can improve your balance skills.

Tips for Starting a Balance Training Program

1. If you plan to start a balance program or any physical activity you have never done before, check with your physician first. Make sure you have no health problems that would make it unsafe for you to participate in the program or activity. Your physician also can recommend specific types of exercises or activities that will be most useful for you.

2. Start any new activity slowly. The first few times you try a new balance program stop *before* you get tired. Over several months you can gradually build up your activity level.

3. It is best to do some sort of balance program at least three times a week to get the most out of it. Remember that it takes time to improve your balance.

Balance Training Programs Outside the Home

Many types of exercise programs may help improve balance. Examples of activities that you can participate in outside the home to improve your balance include dancing, aerobic fitness activities, sports activities, yoga, and Tai Chi.

Dancing

Whether it be square-dancing, doing the polka, or ballroom dancing, all types of dancing can be excellent for your balance. Your local senior center may have information on dance programs in your area.

Aerobic Fitness Programs

Improving your overall level of fitness may help improve your balance. In addition, many adult fitness programs include balance exercises such as standing on one leg and rising up on your toes. You can check with local senior centers to find out about programs in your area.

Be sure to choose a program that is at the right level for you. Many aerobics classes are geared for younger adults and may be too vigorous until you have slowly built up your stamina. Some senior centers and YMCAs offer programs that are specially designed for seniors. If you have not participated in a fitness program before, a senior exercise program is the best place to start.

Sports Activities

Almost any sporting activity will help you with your balance. By participating in sports you learn to make your movements smoother and more precise. Learning these skills may translate to improved balance in everyday activities. Bowling and golf are good examples of sports that can help improve arm and leg coordination. Swimming is another excellent sport for developing coordination.

Yoga

Yoga is a set of exercises where you balance yourself in different body movements and poses. Because the more complex yoga postures can create strain on your joints, you should be sure to start a yoga program slowly by beginning with the simplest stretches first. Yoga classes are offered through YMCAs, adult education classes, and senior centers.

Tai Chi (pronounced Tie Chee)

Tai Chi is a set of exercises where you learn slow, controlled body movements as you move from one position to another. The exercises concentrate on standing balance. A time-honored Eastern tradition, Tai Chi is practiced in China by people of all ages. It recently has become more widespread in the United States. In one study, elderly people who enrolled in Tai Chi classes showed better balance than did other older adults. To find out more about Tai Chi, you can check under "martial arts" in the phone directory.

Balance Activities You Can Do At Home

Exercises that you do at home also can help you improve your balance. Different types of exercises are described in this section. The first type of exercises are done sitting; the second are standing exercises. In general, if you have trouble with your balance, you should start with the sitting exercises and then progress to the standing exercises. If you cannot progress through all of the levels of exercises described, do not be concerned. You will benefit from whatever amount of exercise you can do.

CAUTION: When you try a new exercise, be sure to have someone standing by to help you if you start to fall.

Because the exercises are most difficult the first time you try them, a friend or family member should watch to make sure you are exercising safely.

Sitting Exercises

1. For this type of exercise, you need a straight-backed chair with arms. Sit upright without leaning against the back or arms of the chair with your hands resting in your lap. Keeping your back straight, shift your weight to one side of the chair. Lean over the side of the chair as far as you can without losing your balance, then return to sitting in the center of the chair. Now reverse and lean over the opposite side of the chair in the same fashion. Notice how your body feels when you are upright and balanced. Try to keep this feeling as you shift from side to side.

2. For the next exercise, again sit upright without leaning against the back or arms of the chair. Shift your weight forward as you reach your arms in front of you as far as possible, still keeping your back straight. Now shift your weight back again as you bring your arms back into your lap. Always be careful to keep a straight back. Notice how your body feels when it is upright and balanced (see the illustration on the next page).

Standing Exercises

Tips for Doing Standing Exercises

1. For these exercises you may stand on either a hard floor or carpeting. If the floor is hardwood or linoleum,

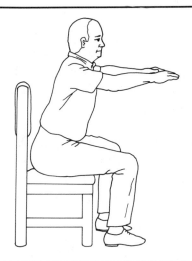

Sitting weight shift forward and back.

make sure it is not slippery. If you are using a carpeted surface, make sure it is not too plush or soft so that you feel unsteady standing on it.

2. Standing exercises should be done wearing sturdy shoes that provide good support. Do not wear shoes with slippery soles or high heels.

3. The first few times you do these exercises you should have someone stand by to make sure you can do them safely on your own. When you first try these exercises, it is also best to hold onto a counter, table top, or sturdy chair for support. As you progress you can start doing the exercises without holding on. Even if you don't hold on, however, you should always stand near something sturdy that you can grab for support if needed.

4. Standing with your back to a corner so that there are walls on each side of you also adds a measure of safety if you start to lose your balance. This also can improve your confidence. To get the full benefit of these exercises, it is very important to do them in a way that makes you feel safe and confident.

5. Hold each of the different standing exercise positions for about 30 seconds if you can. If you cannot hold a particular position that long, do not get discouraged. With practice, your ability to maintain each position gradually will improve.

6. Repeat each exercise at least five times. Remember that improvement comes with lots of practice! Be sure to stop before you get fatigued however. When you get tired your balance is not as good and you will not get as much benefit from the exercises.

7. As you do all of these exercises think of keeping your posture erect with your stomach pulled in and your head up. Maintaining an erect posture will help you keep your balance.

8. Also before you do each exercise, think over in your mind how you are going to do it. Think about how you are going to move with perfect balance, smoothly and precisely. Studies have shown that if you mentally imagine beforehand that you perform an exercise perfectly, your balance improves when you actually do the exercise!

CAUTION: If you have severe neck arthritis, or have problems with dizziness or lightheadedness when you look up, be sure to see your physician before trying any exercise that involves neck or head turning.

Standing on Both Feet

1. Stand with your feet even and close together. With your eyes open, maintain this position. Now close your eyes and again try to keep your balance standing in one place with your feet together.

2. Next, still with your feet close together, move one foot halfway in front of the other foot. Hold this position. Now close your eyes and again hold this position (see the illustration on the next page).

Practice these exercises until you can do them easily. Once you can do these two exercises successfully, you can move on to the next level of balance exercise.

3. Stand with one foot directly in front of the other, both feet pointing straight ahead. First maintain this position with your eyes open, then with your eyes closed (see the illustration on the next page).

After you have mastered these balance exercises try the next three standing exercises.

4. Start with your feet even and close together. Turn your head to one side and up, looking at the ceiling. Feel how you change your balance to continue to stand straight with your head in a different position. Now turn your head to the other side and look up (see the illustration on the next page).

CAUTION: Remember, if you have severe neck arthritis or have problems with dizziness or lightheadedness when you look up, be sure to see your physician before trying any exercise that involves neck or head turning.

A

B

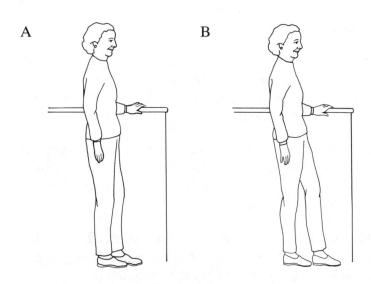

Standing balance: A. One foot halfway in front. B. One foot directly in front.

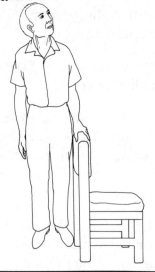

Standing balance with head turned.

5. Now move one foot forward so it is halfway in front of the other foot, just as you did before. Again look first to one side and up, then to the other side and up. Make sure your head movements are slow and smooth.

6. Finally, move one foot completely in front of the other just as you did before. Again look up and to one side and then to the other side and up.

Standing on One Leg

1. Start by holding onto something for support as you stand on one leg. Then try to let go, still keeping your balance on one leg. If you can only hold this position for 1 or 2 seconds to begin with, don't worry. Try to slowly build up to more time. Next, repeat with your other leg. Again do it for as long as you can, up to 20 seconds, and try not to hold onto anything for support.

2. Once you feel comfortable doing a one-leg stand for more than 10 seconds, try standing on one leg with your eyes closed. First try one leg and then the other. Keep your position for as long as possible without holding on.

Bending Down

1. Hold onto a counter top, table, or firm chair for support. Bending your knees a little, reach down as if to pick something up from the floor. Try to go down and come back up as smoothly as you can (see illustration next page).

2. Once you feel comfortable with the exercise, try it without holding onto anything for support. Again, bend down to the floor and straighten back up smoothly and slowly.

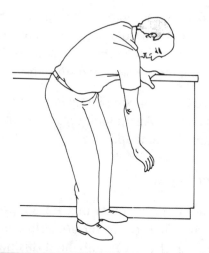

Bending down.

CAUTION: If you get dizzy or lightheaded when you bend down, see your physician before you try this exercise.

Reaching Up

1. Just as for bending down, with this exercise you should also hold onto a table, counter top, or chair. Reach up way over your head as if you were picking fruit off a tree or reaching for a jar off a high shelf. Look up toward where you are reaching. Now bring your arm back to your side.

2. If you feel comfortable doing this exercise, try to reach without holding on for support.

3. Once you have mastered this, try to go up a little onto your tiptoes as you reach. Be sure to hold onto the counter

---

top or table when you first do this. As you become more sure of yourself reaching on tiptoes, try reaching without holding onto anything.

CAUTION: If you have neck arthritis or get dizzy or lightheaded when you look up, remember to see your physician first before you try this exercise.

Braiding Exercises

These exercises are done while standing and moving to the side by sidestepping. Do these exercises along a counter so you can hold onto it if you start to lose your balance. Remember to have someone stand beside you when you are trying these exercises for the first time.

1. Stepping sideways, cross one foot over in front of the other foot. First move to one side going about 20 steps. Then move to the other side, again taking about 20 steps (see illustration next page).

2. Step sideways again, but this time alternate crossing one foot in front of the other and then in back of the other in a braiding fashion. Move about 20 steps in one direction and then repeat moving back the other direction.

Summary

Good balance is the cornerstone of good mobility. Generally older people say their balance is not as good as it was when they were young. Fortunately, balance can be

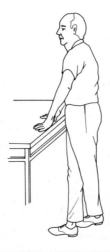

Braiding.

improved with practice. Even if you are only able to do some of the exercises and activities in this chapter, over time you can improve not only your balance, but also your mobility.

Chapter 3

Strengthening Exercises

Strong muscles are essential for staying active! As discussed in Chapter 1, muscle strength is a very important part of balance and mobility. If you have problems with balance, or have impaired mobility, you very likely also have muscle weakness. However, whether you are 60 or 90, with the proper exercise program your muscles *can* get stronger. Improving your muscle strength, regardless of your age, should help both your mobility and your balance.

Several exercises that can be done inside or outside the home that are helpful for older adults with mobility problems are described in this chapter. You do not have to be physically fit to start this exercise program! If you already are quite active, these home exercises still may be appropriate for you. Most of the exercises include a number of more challenging variations. The more difficult exercises are helpful for older adults who are active and trying to maintain or improve their current level of strength and mobility. The goal is to start a safe, yet effective training program to gradually improve your strength, regardless of your current level of physical fitness.

Tips for a Successful Strengthening Program

1. Before starting a new strengthening program, check with your physician to make sure you have no health problems that would prevent you from following an exercise routine. If you have heart disease, high blood pressure, or another chronic medical condition some exercises, such as weight lifting, may be too strenuous for you. However, you still can benefit from other types of strengthening activities such as swimming or a walking program. Your physician can help you select the activity best suited for you.

2. As long as what you are wearing is loose-fitting and comfortable, no special clothing is needed. Be sure not to dress too warmly however. You run the risk of overheating if you work out strenuously and wear clothing which is too heavy.

3. When beginning a new activity, go slow! Do not overdo the number of exercises and stop *before* you develop muscle soreness, not after. Muscles usually do not let you know they have gotten too much of a workout until the next day. For this reason, keep your exercise program very easy the first few times you do it. Gradually, over a period of weeks, you can build up the number of the exercises you do. After that you can increase the level of difficulty of your exercise program.

4. Prior to each exercise session, stretch the muscles you will be strengthening. For instance, if you are doing leg exercises, start with leg stretches. Stretching exercises, which are described in Chapter 5, help to prevent injury and keep you flexible.

5. After you have finished your strengthening exercises, stretch again to "cool down" your muscles. A cool-down period after exercising is very important because older adults can be prone to lightheadedness or even fainting if strengthening exercises are stopped too abruptly. Gentle stretches allow you to gradually slow down after you have finished your strengthening program.

6. Stop exercising if you feel joint or muscle pain while exercising. Slowly and gently start the exercise program over again in a day or two. If you continue to have pain with exercise, you should consult your doctor. The exercises you are doing may not be the right type for you.

CAUTION: If you develop chest pain, lightheadedness, pounding of your heart, or skipped heart beats while you are doing any of these exercises, stop and notify your doctor. You may be experiencing symptoms of a heart condition that your doctor should know about. Your physician can give you guidelines for resuming your strengthening program.

How Often and When to Exercise

One of the keys to successful exercise is finding the best time to do it. Hints on setting up your exercise schedule are provided below.

1. You do not need to repeat your exercise program every day. Every other day should be enough. That way you will give your muscles one day to rest in between workouts.

2. You should avoid exercising for several hours after a full meal. Also be sure not to exercise when you are hungry or thirsty. Working muscles need "fuel" to function at optimal levels.

3. No one time of the day (or night for that matter) is necessarily better to exercise than another. The choice of time to exercise depends on you and your particular schedule. The main thing is to pick a time that will enable you to consistently follow an exercise program.

If you are a "night person" and that is when you have the most energy, you may find exercising in the early evening works out well. If you are a "morning person," in all likelihood you will feel more like exercising in the morning, perhaps before you begin the rest of your day's activities.

Of course, if you are participating in a structured exercise program outside your home, you may need to be flexible and attend a class or participate in an activity when it is offered. Be honest with yourself when starting a new exercise program. Do not join a class or program offered at an inconvenient time for you. Set yourself up for success by choosing an activity that you can follow through with.

4. Do not be too hard on yourself if you don't stick with the first exercise program you try. If one type of activity does not work out for you, try another. Everyone does not enjoy the same types of activities. Again, the main thing is to be active and keep your muscles strong. The specific way you choose to do that is up to you.

Strengthening Exercises You Can Do Outside the Home

Weight Training

Weight-training exercises are designed to stress your muscles by having them do very hard work. When muscles are stressed to near their maximum, they respond by increasing in size. Of course, this affects only the particular muscle that is being worked. Every muscle needs to be specifically trained to increase its size and strength.

Weight-training programs can be done at any age. However, if you have heart disease, high blood pressure, or other chronic medical conditions, your physician may recommend that you see a physical therapist for an exercise prescription before starting a weight-training program. By monitoring your heart while your muscle strength is being tested, the therapist can determine what weights you can safely tolerate.

Weight-training programs are offered at many gymnasiums and health clubs. If your physician feels you can safely begin weight-training without medical guidance, check to see if a program near you has trained staff members who can help you start on a schedule using weights appropriate for your needs.

Swimming

Swimming is excellent exercise for strengthening both your arms and legs. It allows you to grade the amount of resistance your muscles work against by varying how hard you pull through the water. In addition, swimming can be a very gentle exercise and is usually well tolerated. If you have arthritis, swimming may be the best type of exercise for you because it does not put a great deal of strain on your joints.

Group Fitness Programs

Many adult fitness programs include strengthening exercises as part of their activities. Some programs use light ankle or wrist weights during the workout. Special classes for seniors frequently are offered through YMCAs, local senior centers, schools, or hospitals.

Strengthening Exercises You Can Do At Home

This section describes a number of exercises you can do at home to strengthen various muscles that are important for good balance and mobility. Some of the exercises specifically target buttock and abdominal muscles. Other exercises are designed to strengthen your thigh or lower leg muscles.

You should do at least one type of exercise for each muscle group. When you do these exercises, finish working one muscle group before going on to the next. Remember to do a few stretches (see Chapter 5) before and after your strengthening exercises.

How to Choose Your Level of Exercise Difficulty

The exercises in this section are designed to be appropriate for older adults who have muscle weakness or problems with mobility. At the same time, if you are already quite physically active, these exercises can be adapted so that they provide a good workout for you. You can make each exercise more difficult by increasing the number of times you do it or by increasing the amount of time you hold each strengthening position. Many of the exercises also can be made more difficult by using weights.

As a general rule, first increase the number of times that you do each exercise, then increase the amount of time that you hold each exercise position. Once you have reached the maximum guidelines for repetitions and holding time, move on to the more difficult version of the exercise or add weights so the exercise provides you a good workout.

Velcro wrist and ankle weights are sold in many sporting goods and department stores. The lightest ones, which you should start with, are 1/2 to 1 pound. You also can make simple ankle weights by putting sand in a small cloth bag and draping it over your ankle.

If You Have Muscle Weakness

If you are not sure whether you have weak leg muscles, see the section "Testing Your Muscle Strength" in Chapter 1, page 13, for a simple test of your baseline level of muscle strength. Start each exercise in its most basic form. If you have weak leg muscles, the beginning level of exercise most likely will be the right amount of difficulty for you. Continue doing each exercise at the lowest number of repetitions until it becomes very comfortable for you. Only then should you start slowly increasing the number of repetitions. Once you have increased the number of times you do each exercise, slowly increase the amount of time each exercise position is held. Remember you never want to work at a level that feels extremely difficult to you. You want to advance in difficulty only when the level you are doing has become very easy for you.

If You Do Not Have Muscle Weakness

If you do not have muscle weakness, or if you are already physically active, you still should start with the basic exercises. If you find these exercises are not at all difficult, you can advance rapidly over a few days to a higher number of repetitions and then to a longer holding time for each position. When you have advanced to doing the maximum number of repetitions for the maximum amount of time, and an exercise still is not difficult for you, move on to the more difficult version or add weights when doing the exercise.

When you reach a stage of exercise where it feels moderately, but not extremely, difficult, you have found your appropriate workout level. From this point, you should advance more slowly, moving to the next level only when you feel the exercise you are doing has become very comfortable and easy.

Exercising Your Back and Buttocks

These muscles are essential for stabilizing your back and pelvis whenever you start to lose and then regain your balance, for example, when you start to fall but catch yourself. Your buttock muscles also are important for climbing hills and stairs. When you first begin these exercises, choose just one of the three listed below. As you become stronger, you can build up to doing all three.

Bridging

To do this exercise, lie down on a bed or the floor on your back with your knees bent and your feet flat. If you are uncomfortable, you can place pillows under your back and neck for comfort. From this starting position, raise your hips off the surface several inches by tightening your buttock muscles. You should feel your seat muscles tighten as you raise your pelvis. Hold this position for a few seconds, then slowly and smoothly lower your hips back down to the floor or bed (see the illustration below). Repeat twice to start.

Slowly build up, as tolerated, until you can do the exercise 10 times. You also can increase the amount of time you hold the hips-up position up to 10 seconds.

Gluteal Sets

This exercise can be done either standing or lying on your back. With your back straight in a comfortable position, squeeze your buttocks together. Hold your seat muscles tight for a count of five, then relax. Repeat twice. Gradually

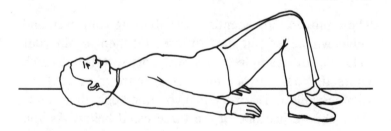

Bridging.

add a couple more gluteal sets to your exercise sessions until you build up to a total of 10 repetitions.

Back Leg Lifts

Find a counter top or sturdy chair for support to do this exercise. Stand behind the chair or counter top and grasp it firmly with both hands. Shift your weight to one leg and slowly raise your other leg straight out behind you. Keep both knees straight as you do this. Hold your leg up behind you for a count of three, then slowly lower it back to the ground (see illustration below). Repeat several times with the same leg. Then switch legs and repeat several times with the opposite leg.

Gradually increase the number of repetitions you do up to 8 to 10 on each side. You then can increase the diffi-

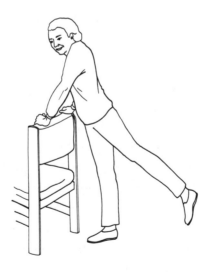

Back leg lifts.

culty of this exercise by increasing the amount of time you hold your leg up. Try to hold your leg up for a few more seconds each time until you can hold it up for 10 seconds at a time. You also can work on lifting your leg higher behind you. Remember to keep your posture as erect as possible while you are lifting your leg behind you.

Another way to make this exercise more difficult is to use velcro weights around your ankles or to wear heavy shoes. If you would like to try a weight, start with just one pound of resistance and gradually increase in one pound increments.

Exercising Your Abdomen

This exercise works on your abdominal muscles. These muscles are extremely important for your balance because they function as a brace to keep your back stable.

Partial Sit Up

Start by lying on your back with your knees bent, keeping your feet flat on the floor or bed. Cross your hands over your chest. Tighten your abdominal muscles and slowly curl forward to lift your shoulder blades off the floor or bed. Keep your neck straight as you curl yourself up and do a partial sit up. Hold this position for several seconds then slowly and smoothly lie back down (see illustration on the next page).

When you do this exercise, be careful not to pull up too far off the floor. You only need to raise up several inches, or just enough to lift your shoulder blades off the floor or bed. Also remember to keep your arms relaxed as you do

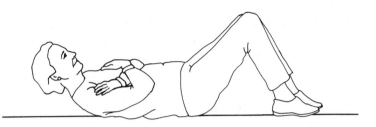

Partial sit ups.

the exercise. Your lower back should be firmly pressed into the bed or floor. Finally, continue to breathe as you do your partial sit up. It may take some practice, but you can continue to breath normally while you tighten your stomach muscles.

When you first start, you should do this exercise only two or three times. You can gradually build up to doing 10 repetitions. You also can increase, up to 10 seconds, the amount of time you hold the curled-up position.

This is one of the more difficult exercises described. If you cannot lift yourself high enough to clear your shoulder blades when you first start, do not be discouraged. Many people have fairly weak stomach muscles when they start an exercise program. However, these muscles gradually will become stronger as you continue your strengthening program.

CAUTION: If you have severe osteoporosis or compression fractures in your back (see Chapter 9), you should *not* do this exercise. Doing a partial sit up increases the pressure on the front part of the bones in your back. If you already have severe osteoporosis, this exercise may increase the risk of developing a compression fracture.

Exercising Your Abdomen and Thighs

In addition to strengthening your abdominal muscles, these exercises also increase thigh strength. Thigh muscle strength is important for climbing stairs or hills and for getting out of a chair or bed. Thigh muscles also play a key role in maintaining your knee stability and preventing your knees from giving way.

Straight-Leg Raise

Lie on a flat surface with one knee bent and the other leg straight. Your arms should be relaxed and down at your sides. Lock the knee of your straight leg by tightening the muscle on the top of your thigh. Then raise that leg up about 12 inches, being sure to keep the knee straight. Hold your leg up for a few seconds, then lower it slowly back down to resting position, again being certain to keep your knee locked (see illustration on the next page). Repeat once more, then do two repetitions with the opposite leg. By keeping one leg bent as you exercise the other leg, you are stabilizing your back and keeping it flat on the bed or floor. As your stomach and thigh muscles get stronger, you gradually can increase the number of leg raises you do, up to 10 on each side. Also, as this exercise gets easier, you can start increasing the amount of time you hold the leg in a raised position. Try to work up to 5 seconds.

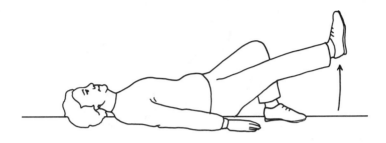

Straight leg raise.

A more difficult version of this exercise is to use a 1 to 2 pound weight on your ankles or wear shoes to add resistance when you exercise. Remember the key is to keep the knee of the leg you are lifting straight! If you notice your knee is bending, go back to doing an easier version of the exercise.

Sit Squats

Beside the abdomen and thigh muscles, this exercise also works your buttock muscles. Find a sturdy chair that is about knee height or a little taller. Cross your arms in front of your chest as you stand in front of the chair. Keeping your back straight, slowly and smoothly lower yourself into the chair, then slowly and smoothly stand back up again without uncrossing your arms (see illustration on the next page).

If you find this exercise difficult, try a higher chair. When you are stronger, switch back to a lower chair. At first, do just two or three repetitions. As you build up your strength, you gradually can increase the number of repetitions you do up to 10.

This exercise can be made more challenging by using lower and lower chairs. You also can slow down the

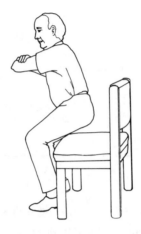

Sit squats.

---

speed with which you sit and stand. This will make your muscles work harder as well.

Exercising Your Thighs

Your thigh muscles are the largest muscles in your body. Keeping them strong is critical to remaining active and mobile.

Side Leg Lifts

Find a sturdy chair with a high back. Stand behind the chair and firmly grasp the top of the chair with both hands. Stand comfortably with both feet pointing toward the chair. Slowly lift one leg out to the side and raise it several inches off the floor. Be sure to keep your foot

---

pointing forward as you lift your leg. Hold this position for a few seconds, then lower your leg back to the floor (see illustration below). Repeat this exercise twice with each leg. Gradually build up to doing 8 or 10 leg lifts on each side.

You also can gradually increase the length of time you hold the leg lift up to 10 seconds with each leg. Once you feel comfortable holding each lift for 10 seconds, start raising your leg higher. This exercise also can be done using a 1 to 2 pound ankle weight to increase the degree of difficulty.

Kicks

Sit in a sturdy, comfortable chair that has good back support. Straighten one leg out in front of you, making sure

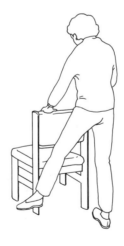

Side leg lifts.

the knee is completely straight. Hold this position for a few seconds then relax (see illustration below). Repeat several times with each leg.

As your strength improves, increase the number of kicks up to 10 times on each side. Then increase the time you hold each leg straight, up to 10 seconds. Once you feel comfortable with this version of the exercise for 10 repetitions on each side, you can continue to strengthen your upper legs by putting weights around your ankles. You should start with just 1 or 2 pounds, but you gradually can increase up to as much weight as is comfortable for you.

Exercising Your Lower Leg Muscles

Your lower leg muscles are very important for walking and climbing hills. These muscles also help you catch

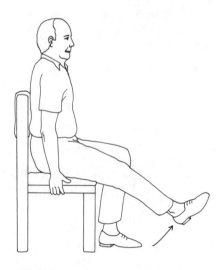

Kicks.

yourself if you begin to fall. If you have trouble with balance, it is especially important for you to keep these muscles strong.

Standing on Tiptoe

For this exercise hold onto the top of a high-backed sturdy chair or counter top with both hands for support. Raise up onto both tiptoes, making sure you are standing up straight as you do this. Remain up on your toes for a few seconds, then come back down (see the illustration top of next page). Do this exercise 3 times. You gradually can increase to 10 times and hold the tiptoe position for up to 10 seconds.

Foot Lifts

For this exercise sit in a sturdy chair with both feet flat on the floor. Raise up the ball and toes of one foot as far as you can, keeping your heel on the floor. Hold this position for 2 to 3 seconds, then lower your foot back to the floor. Remember to keep your heel on the ground while you are doing this exercise (see the illustration bottom of next page). Repeat several times on each side.

As you get stronger, increase the number of repetitions to 10 times on each side. Then increase the amount of time that you hold your foot in the "up" position to a maximum of 10 seconds for each trial.

When you feel comfortable doing 10 repetitions, holding each for 10 seconds, you can try doing this exercise with weights on your foot. Take an ankle weight or a sand-

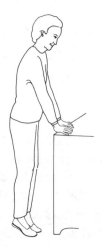

Standing on tiptoe.

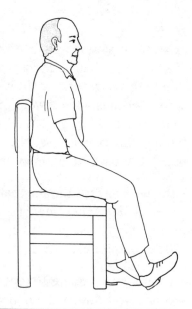

Foot lifts.

filled bag and place it over your foot. Place the weight as far out on your foot as you can and repeat the exercise. Be sure to keep your heel on the floor. If you use weights, start with 1 pound and then gradually increase up to about 5 pounds.

Summary

Some of the most important exercises for older adults are those that build strength. If you are healthy and mobile, strengthening activities or exercises are essential for maintaining an active lifestyle. If your mobility is impaired, strengthening exercises will play a crucial role for you in preventing further loss of function and independence. By performing the activities or exercises described in this chapter, you may not just stabilize but actually improve your overall level of mobility and function!

Chapter 4

Posture

Changes in Posture With Age

To a certain extent, changes in body alignment are a common part of aging. As you get older your posture tends to become slightly more curved. This small change in posture is due to normal alterations in the bones and joints of your back, hips, and knees (see the illustration below).

Changes in Your Back

Your back has a natural S-shaped curve which becomes a little more exaggerated as you get older. Your head is at the top of the "S" and moves slightly forward with age. The other curves in your upper and lower back also become slightly more pronounced with age, resulting in a rounded upper back and shoulders, and a swayed lower back.

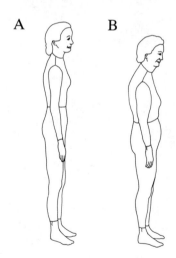

Posture changes with age: A. Young adult. B. Older adult

Much of this change in back posture is due to alterations in the joints in your back. The joints between the vertebrae, or bones of your back, are composed of spongy cushions called discs. Collagen, a protein that is very elastic, makes up a large part of these discs and is very important for keeping them springy. Because collagen gets stiffer as you get older, over time your discs naturally lose some of their spring and flatten out. As the discs flatten, you tend to get shorter, and the curvature of your spine becomes more exaggerated.

Changes in Your Hips and Knees

Many older people stay a little bent at the hips and knees when they stand. Changes in collagen as you age predispose you to this alteration in body posture. As the collagen in your body stiffens, it gets harder for you to completely stretch out the muscles and joints in your legs. However, more often than not, it is a decreased activity level, in combination with collagen changes, that causes the flexed position of your hips and knees. When you sit or lie in a curled-up position for long periods of time, some of the muscles in your legs shorten, and the hip and knee joints stiffen. This makes it harder for you to straighten the knees and hips fully when you stand up.

Is Poor Posture An Inevitable Part Of Aging?

Changes in postures with aging are not inevitable. Everyone has seen someone who, even at the age of 80 or 90, has a very straight back and erect posture. Just because you are older, you should not expect to have a marked curvature of the spine or a stooped, bent over appearance.

On the other hand, some older people have quite dramatic changes in posture. Severe changes in body alignment are related to conditions that are not necessarily a normal part of aging. Problems with osteoporosis can cause you to have a more curved back. A stooped, bent over appearance also may be due to the loss of flexibility that results if you decrease your activity level.

How Osteoporosis Affects Your Posture

The bones of your back may be weakened by osteoporosis (see Chapter 9). When osteoporosis is severe enough, some of the vertebrae actually may crumble. This will cause you to have more of a curve in your upper back as the vertebrae collapse on themselves.

How Loss of Flexibility Affects Your Posture

Many people, both old and young, tend to sit for long periods of time. Prolonged sitting may increase the curve in the upper back and contribute to a stooped posture. When sitting, most people tend to relax the muscles holding their back upright, and as a result, they hunch forward. Sitting with a curved upper back position for a long time can make the muscles and joints of your back less flexible. As the stiffness in your back increases, it becomes harder for you to fully straighten up.

Why Is Good Posture So Important?

Making Your Muscles Work Efficiently

If you have poor posture, walking and getting around will be harder for you to do. This is because your muscles for walking work best when your body is in good alignment. When your body alignment is poor, your muscles have to work harder to do their job.

Preventing Back Pain

Poor posture also can lead to pain in your muscles, particularly those in the back and neck. Sometimes this pain comes and goes; at other times it can become persistent. Doing exercises to straighten your neck and back can help relieve the muscle pain associated with poor posture. Chapter 5 contains a number of good neck and back stretching exercises.

Preventing Leg and Back Stiffness

Poor posture not only can lead to back pain, but it also can increase back and leg stiffness. As your legs and back get stiffer, your posture may become more bent and stooped. Poor posture leads to even poorer posture. Erect posture, on the other hand, helps you keep your flexibility. At the same time, maintaining your flexibility also helps preserve good posture.

Preventing Compression Fractures

Poor posture can increase the likelihood of damaging the bones in your back. When you sit hunched forward, the bones in your back are under more pressure than when you are sitting up straight. A slumped forward posture increases the weight on the front part of the bones in your back. If the weight increases too much, and if your bones are already weakened because of osteoporosis, the front part of the vertebrae may actually break. These breaks are called compression fractures. An erect posture eliminates excessive stress on the front on the vertebrae and decreases the likelihood of compression fractures.

How To Check For Good Posture

To check for good standing posture, position yourself with your back to a wall and your heels 2 inches away. If you have erect posture, you should have three points of contact with the wall: (1) the back of your head, (2) your shoulder blades, and (3) your buttocks. There should be only enough room between the small of your back and the wall for your flattened hand to fit. Notice how your legs feel as you stand there. If you have erect posture you will be able to completely straighten your knees in this standing position (see the illustration on the next page).

If you cannot get your head or shoulder blades to touch the wall, you probably have too large of a curve in your upper back. Although part of this exaggerated curve may be due to changes in your back that you cannot reverse, some improvement can be achieved by working on your posture.

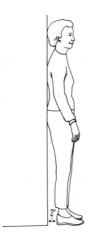

Checking for good posture.

If you cannot straighten your legs completely when you stand close to the wall, you may have a problem with joint stiffness in your knees and hips. Often much of this joint stiffness can be decreased by working on your posture and flexibility. Ways to achieve good posture are discussed in more detail in the next section.

Achieving Good Posture

Remembering to always sit and stand straight is the most important thing you can do to keep good posture. It also is important to pay attention to maintaining an erect posture in all positions, including lying down, and in all movements, especially bending and lifting.

Good Standing Posture

Begin by standing against a wall with your heels 2 inches away as you did when you were checking your posture (see the illustration on page 57). Remember you should try to have the back of your head, your shoulder blades, and your buttocks all making contact with the wall.

1. Now try to place your flattened hand between the small of your back and the wall. If your hand can move easily behind the small of your back, tighten your buttock muscles and try to flatten your lower back against the wall. Tightening your seat muscles will decrease the amount of sway in your lower back and help you achieve a more erect position.

2. Next note if your head is touching the wall. If your head does not touch the wall, try a "chin tuck" to move your head back. Move your whole neck back toward the wall, making sure your head is straight and not tipped back.

3. Finally, notice your hips and knees. Try to straighten them as much as possible, while still keeping your head, shoulders, and buttocks touching the wall.

If you have compression fractures or long-standing postural abnormalities, you may not be able to achieve all three points of contact. Regardless of how well you are able to do this activity, it still can be a valuable exercise for improving your posture.

As you are doing these exercises, try to make a mental image of how it feels to be standing as straight as you can. Remember this image when you are standing. Make yourself as erect as possible whenever you are standing, just as if you were practicing with a wall behind you.

Good Sitting Posture

It is easiest to achieve an erect sitting posture if you use chairs that are firm and have good back support. Ideally, all the furniture you sit on would be designed for your body's exact size and shape. Of course, this is not the case, so you need to be aware of your sitting posture. Paying attention to how you sit will help you achieve the most optimal body alignment, no matter what type of chair you find yourself using.

Tips on Good Sitting Posture

1. To achieve a good sitting posture, the first thing you need to do is to position yourself with your buttocks as far back in the seat as possible. A very common mistake is to sit with the buttocks positioned forward in the chair. This results in a slouched posture with a rounded lower back and puts increased pressure on the front of your vertebrae.

2. Keep your shoulders straight and relaxed against the back of the chair. Remember, whenever you are sitting, to keep your shoulders back and your spine erect. This includes when you are riding in a car or driving, as well as when you are attending a concert or show.

3. Your chin should stay upright with your head level and facing forward to keep your neck in erect alignment.

4. There should be a slight space between the small of your back and the chair. A thin pillow placed behind the small of the back can give support to the lower back and maintain the normal curve in your spine (see the illustration on the next page).

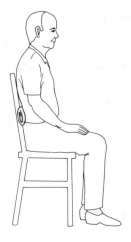

Good sitting posture.

Small round pillows designed to provide extra back support (lumbar rolls) are available in many medical supply stores. However, some people may find these too firm. You may need to experiment with various sizes, and different types of materials, to find a cushion that is comfortable for you. A homemade back support can be made quite easily by rolling up a small bath towel and securing it with tape.

Good Posture When Lying Down

Maintaining correct posture also is important when you are lying down. Considering how much time is spent in lying positions, compared to the amount of time spent up

---

and moving around, it is very important to pay attention to your posture when lying down.

1. Lying on your back can be uncomfortable if your lower back does not get enough support. If it is uncomfortable for you to lie flat on your back, try lying with your legs slightly elevated, supported by a pillow under your calves. This will take the stress off of your lower spine.

2. Change positions every several hours during the night. People often do this without ever waking up. Remaining in one position for longer than about 2 hours can cause your joints to become stiff and uncomfortable. For correct posture you need to be especially aware not to stay in a curled up position for long periods of time.

3. If you notice discomfort in your back or hips when you are lying on your side, it may be because your pelvis is excessively tilted. If it is uncomfortable for you to lie on your side, try bending your knees and hips and placing a soft, thin pillow between your legs. This will help straighten your pelvis.

4. Make sure that you are sleeping on a firm surface. A mattress that is too soft will give an abnormal curvature to the spine, increasing the strain on your back muscles. A firm mattress or a firm waterbed is recommended for maintaining good posture. One simple way to make your bed firmer is to place a plywood board between the mattress and box springs. Often this is all you need to give your back adequate support.

Stretching Exercises To Improve Posture

If you have trouble with your posture, chances are you need to improve your flexibility as well. Joint and muscle stiffness makes it harder for you to completely straighten out and achieve erect posture.

Moving around is the key to staying flexible. When you are sitting, straighten your legs frequently and stand up and stretch as often as you can. Also, when you are lying down, you need to remember to stretch out frequently. It is especially important to be sure you are not always in a curled-up position.

Exercises that improve your flexibility also will help improve your posture. Stretching exercises for the muscles around the knees and hips will help you straighten these joints completely when you stand. Back and trunk stretching exercises will loosen the muscles of the back and may help improve back alignment.

Chapter 5 describes a number of back and leg exercises designed to increase your flexibility. The Hamstring Stretch described in that chapter (see page 78) is particularly good for posture. If you have trouble straightening your knees when you stand, this may be a very helpful stretching exercise for you.

Two other exercises for posture are described below. One is good for straightening the upper back. The other exercise helps to straighten out the hips.

Upper Back Stretch

You may do this exercise either standing or sitting. If you are sitting, use a firm chair. With your elbows bent, and keeping your shoulders down, pull your shoulder blades back and together. Tuck in your chin and keep your head up straight as you do this. Hold your position for 5 seconds, then relax (see the illustration top of next page). Repeat this stretch five times.

Hip Stretch

Stand facing a dresser, sturdy chair, or counter top that you can hold onto for support. Stand with your weight on one leg. Place the other leg behind you, with the knee bent, resting your toes on the floor. Now, keeping your trunk as erect as possible, slowly straighten your back knee. You should feel a stretch in the front of the thigh and hip of that leg. Hold this position for 5 seconds, then bend your knee again (see the illustration bottom of next page). Repeat this stretch five times with each leg.

Summary

Although some changes in posture may not be reversible, much can be done to straighten your body's alignment. Being aware of how you stand, sit, and lie is the key to improving your posture. Stretching your muscles and joints also will help you maintain an erect posture. As you work on improving your posture, you should find that your mobility improves as well!

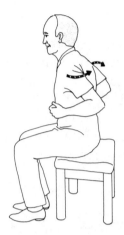

Upper back stretch.

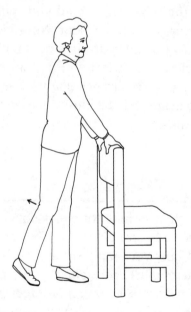

Hip stretch.

Chapter 5

Flexibility and Stretching Exercises

Changes in Flexibility With Age

All people become less flexible as they get older. Think of how limber a child is compared to people in their 40s, compared to people in their 80s. It is normal for your body to become stiffer as you age. There are two main reasons for this. One is because of a change in a body protein called collagen. The other is because people tend to move around less as they get older. Both of these reasons are discussed in more detail below.

The Role of Collagen

Body tissues that allow flexibility, such as muscles, tendons, connective tissues, and cartilage, tighten as you age. All of these tissues contain a protein called collagen. This protein is a very elastic, springy material, and without it you would not be able to move at all. As you age, the fibers of collagen move closer together and stick to each other. As a result, the tissues in your body become less elastic and less flexible.

It is easiest to see the effects of these collagen changes on your skin in the form of wrinkles. Partly because of the change in collagen, your skin loses its elasticity and wrinkles more as you get older. These changes also happen to collagen in other parts of the body.

Joints, in particular, depend on collagen to stay mobile. This is true not only of the knee, hip, and ankle joints, but also of all the joints between each of the bones in the back. The increased stiffness of collagen is part of the reason your back becomes less flexible as you get older.

The Role of Activity

"Use it or lose it" is a saying everyone has heard. This expression explains much of what aging is all about. In general, you need to be physically active to stay flexible. If you stop being active, you will lose some of your flexibility.

Many people have had the unfortunate experience of breaking a bone. When the cast is removed after several weeks, the joint is much harder to move. Immobilization, whether it is because of a cast or a long period of bed rest, can cause your joints to stiffen up. In fact, if you do not regularly move your joints to the fullest extent possible, they will tend to tighten and lose some of their flexibility. For example, if you do not regularly reach over your head, as when getting things down from high cupboards or shelves, your shoulder may "freeze" somewhat. If this happens, when you do try to reach over your head, your shoulder won't be limber enough to extend as far as it used to.

Why Is Good Flexibility So Important?

Ability to Move Smoothly

Good flexibility is essential for several reasons. First of all, you must be limber to be able to move around easily. The stiffness that occurs with aging affects your ability to move smoothly. Think of how a young person walks, using a lot of arm swing and trunk movement. This requires flexibility. When you are older, walking becomes more rigid with a decrease in arm swing and less trunk movement with each step.

Maintaining Mobility

If you have lost your flexibility, you will not be as mobile as you would like, simply because of stiffness. When your body feels stiff, it becomes harder for you to walk. This stiffness may cause you to walk in a way that is unnatural and awkward. When you walk with a rigid gait, you use up much more energy than if you walk with a normal gait. As a result, you won't be able to walk as far before you become fatigued.

Maintaining Good Posture

Flexibility also is important for maintaining good posture. When you lose flexibility, it becomes harder for you to straighten your joints completely. The more stiffness you have, the more likely you are to be bent forward when you stand. Chapter 4 describes in greater detail how loss of flexibility affects your posture.

Achieving Flexibility

Even though your tissues naturally get stiffer with age, they can still stretch. As an older person, you can gain flexibility just as a younger person can. Working on your flexibility now will help guarantee that you stay active and fit in the future.

Increase Your Activity

Being active today is the key to staying active tomorrow! Most kinds of physical activities will help keep you limber. Whatever the activity, be it housework, gardening, dancing, or simply walking, the more you move around, the more you will be able to stay flexible.

Specific Activities to Increase Flexibility

Some types of activities are ideally suited for increasing flexibility.

1. Many fitness classes for seniors include specific stretching exercises both at the beginning and the end of the exercise period.

2. Swimming provides a good stretching workout. Although this sport is especially good for the arms and upper body, the frog kick in particular helps work on leg flexibility.

3. Yoga also is an excellent activity for increasing flexibility. Using a slow, smooth approach to movement, yoga works on all parts of your body, not just one area.

Specific Ways to Increase Flexibility at Home

Even if you are limited in mobility and cannot participate in exercise classes, swimming, or yoga, your joints still will benefit from any increase in activity. Older people need to stand up, walk around, lift their arms, and straighten their legs frequently. When you are sitting down, try to change positions frequently. Shift your weight in the chair every 15 minutes or so, and stand up and stretch if you have been sitting for an hour at a time.

When lying down, also change positions frequently. It is especially important not to lie curled-up for long periods of time, because this position increases knee and hip stiffness. Be sure to stretch your legs all the way out from time to time.

Stretches You Can Do Routinely During the Day

One excellent way to increase flexibility is to stretch your joints routinely throughout the day. For example, you can do simple stretches while you are reading or watching television. There are a number of back, leg, and ankle stretches you can do easily while you're relaxing in your favorite chair.

1. Stretch your back several times a day by bending forward and straightening and by twisting first to one side and then to the other.

2. Straighten your legs, one at a time, in front of you.

3. Pump your ankles up and down, both when your legs are bent and when they are straight.

4. Move your feet around in circles, first in one direction and then in the opposite direction.

The following Dos and Don'ts of Stretching will help you let your body be your guide as to how far you can safely stretch.

Dos and Don'ts of Stretching

After following a stretching program for several weeks, you will find that you are more limber and able to stretch farther. Regardless of your age, you can safely start a home stretching program to increase your flexibility. However, you need to follow a few simple precautions.

1. When you start your stretching program, do not over-stretch. Go as far as you can in a stretch, but not to the point of pain. Stop where you feel a comfortable tightness in your muscles or joints.

2. Stretching needs to be done slowly! When you get to your maximum stretch, stay there for 10 to 30 seconds. As you age, your joints, muscles, and ligaments require more time to stretch than they did when you were younger. By doing stretches slowly, the collagen has time to lengthen.

3. Stretching needs to be done consistently. To keep your collagen as elastic as possible, you should stretch every day.

4. Stretching should be done smoothly. Don't bounce! You may think you are increasing your stretch by bouncing, but in fact, you may cause your tissues to tear. This can make you less, rather than more, flexible.

5. Remember to stretch all parts of your body, not just your legs. To keep as limber as possible, you need to stretch your neck, shoulders, arms, and back in addition to your hips and legs.

CAUTION: If you have neck arthritis, or if you have ever fainted or gotten dizzy when tilting your head back, check with your physician before you do the neck exercises. The vertebrae and blood supply through your neck area are at risk of injury if you have these problems.

Specific Stretching Exercises

Repeat each of the following stretching exercises two to five times, holding each stretch for 10 to 30 seconds.

Stretching Exercises for Your Neck

You may do these exercises either sitting or standing.

Head Turns

Turn your head slowly to one side and look behind your shoulder as far as you can. Hold your head position for at least 10 seconds. You should feel a gentle stretch in your neck muscles as you do this. Now turn your head to the other side and look over the other shoulder (see the illustration on the next page).

Head Tilts

Start by looking straight ahead. Now bend your head to one side, bringing your ear towards your shoulder. You should feel a gentle stretch in the muscles in the side of your neck. Keep your shoulders down and relaxed as you hold the stretch. Now bend your head to the other side (see the illustration on the next page).

Stretching Exercises for Your Shoulders and Arms

As with the neck exercises, you can exercise your shoulders and arms while either sitting or standing.

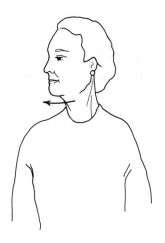

Head turns.

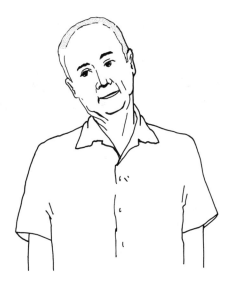

Head tilts.

Forward Reaches

Extend both arms out in front of you. Keeping your back straight, reach out as far forward as possible (see the illustration below). This exercise can be done with both arms together or each arm separately if you find that more comfortable.

Overhead Stretch

Reach both arms up over your head as far as possible. If you find one arm stretches farther than the other, clasp your hands together as you reach overhead. In this way the more flexible arm can help stretch the tighter one.

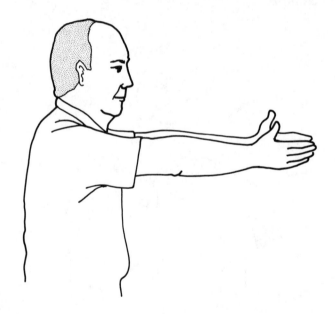

Forward reach.

Shoulder Shrugs

Bring your shoulders up toward your ears. Hold for a count of 10. Relax. You can try this exercise one shoulder at a time if that feels easier.

Stretching Exercises for Your Trunk

Trunk Twists

This exercise helps stretch your neck and shoulders as well as your back. Start from a sitting position. Place your hands on your shoulders. Keeping your elbows out to the sides, twist your head, neck, and trunk as a unit to one side. Go as far as you comfortably can. You should feel the stretch in your upper back. Next, still keeping your hands on your shoulders, twist to the other side. When you do this exercise, try not to swivel your knees as you twist your upper back (see the illustration below).

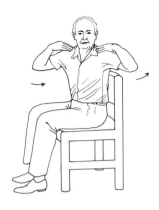

Trunk twists.

Back Extension

Sit on a firm chair with your feet supported on the floor and your hands relaxed in your lap. Pretend there is a string attached to the top of your head that is being pulled to lift you up. Keeping your head up, straighten your back and, at the same time, bring your shoulders back (see the illustration below).

Stretching Exercises for your Hips and Back

Hip Rolls

For this exercise you will need to lie down, either on the floor or on a firm bed. Bend your knees up, keeping your

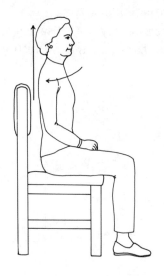

Back extension.

feet flat on the surface and your knees together. Roll your knees to one side as far as possible. Come back to the middle so your knees again are pointing straight up. Then roll to the other side as far as you can (see the illustration below).

Knee to Chest

Lie down with your legs straight. Bring one leg up toward your chest as far as you can by bending your knee and hip. Then lower your leg back down and repeat with the other leg (see the illustration below).

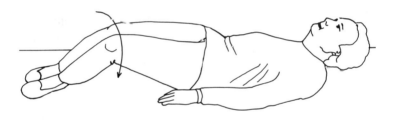

Hip rolls.

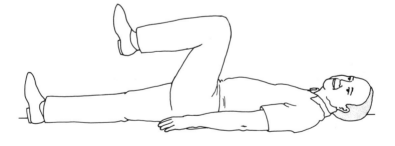

Knee to chest.

Stretching Exercises for Your Legs

Hamstring Stretch

For this exercise you should be sitting in a chair. With your knee straight, elevate one leg on a small footstool. The other leg should be bent with your foot flat on the floor. Place both hands on the knee resting on the footstool. Now lean forward from the waist, feeling the stretch in the back of your knee. Next change legs and again lean forward to stretch your other hamstring muscle (see the illustration below).

Calf Stretch

Stand up and hold onto a counter or the back of a chair for support. Place one foot forward in front of the other. Push

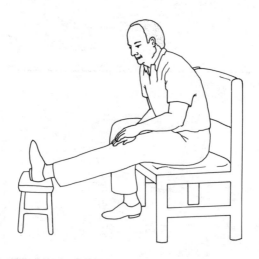

Hamstring stretch.

your hips forward and bend the front knee slightly, keeping the back heel flat on the floor. You should feel the stretch in the calf muscles of your back leg. Now switch legs and repeat the stretch (see the illustration below).

Stretching Exercise for Your Ankles

Ankle Circles

This exercise can be done either sitting or lying down. Make slow circles with the ankle. Keeping your leg still, circle your foot all the way around in one direction, then reverse and circle the other direction. Repeat with the other ankle (see the illustration on the next page).

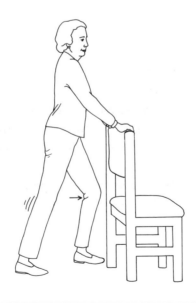

Calf stretch.

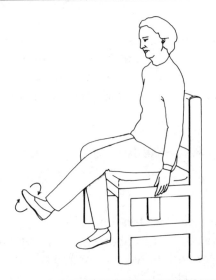

Ankle circles.

Summary

Being flexible allows you to be as mobile as possible. Although it does get harder to stay limber as you grow older, it is not impossible. With a good stretching program, you can prevent your joints from becoming stiff. With time and effort, you may gain back some of the suppleness you had when you were younger.

Chapter 6

Circulation and Heart Conditioning

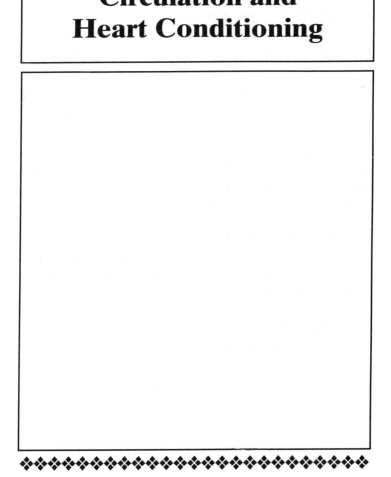

Your mobility depends not only on your posture, strength, and flexibility, but also on your circulation and the ability of your heart to pump blood to your muscles. Circulation plays a key role in determining how much work or exercise you can do. Your ability to walk or do any other activity depends on the ability of your heart to pump blood to your body tissues.

Changes in Your Heart and Circulation with Age

If you are a healthy, active older adult, chances are that when you are resting and not exerting yourself your heart still pumps just as efficiently as it did when you were young. However, as you get older your heart rate will not increase as much with exercise as it did when you were young. This change should not affect your mobility, except in situations where you have to work exceptionally hard, such as climbing several flights of stairs or walking up a long steep hill.

Even though your heart rate does not speed up as much, if you are physically fit, you still can do quite strenuous activities. It is not that rare to see older adults participate in competitive sports.

A decline in physical function used to be considered normal aging. It is now known, as a general rule, that this is not true. With a consistent level of exercise and activity, it is possible to keep the heart and circulatory systems working efficiently throughout the life span.

Conditioning Level and Medical Problems

Why can some older people still run marathons while others cannot climb a flight of stairs? There are many reasons for this. Two of the most important factors are the individual's overall "conditioning" level and whether he or she has major medical problems, especially heart disease.

Level of Conditioning

Many older adults are not as physically active as they were when they were young. Lack of good conditioning, or being out of shape, is one of the major reasons why older people lose their mobility.

Good body conditioning means being physically fit. It means your heart pumps strongly and you have good circulation. Good conditioning also means that your body tissues, especially your muscles, are efficient in using the oxygen and other nutrients delivered in the blood. When you are physically fit, you are able to do strenuous exercise because your heart, circulation, and muscles all function at maximum capacity.

If you have been active all of your life, you are more likely to have good conditioning as you get older. If you have been physically inactive most of your life, your overall level of conditioning may not be as good.

If you are "out of shape," even though your heart still pumps fine when you are quietly sitting, when you are up and moving around your heart may not pump as well as it should. Also, your muscles will not work as efficiently. As a result, you will tire easily. For example, if you are in good shape, you can walk at a brisk pace without getting tired or out of breath. If you are not in such good shape, however, walking rapidly may be quite difficult for you.

Medical Problems

Another reason people become less energetic and mobile as they grow older is because they have chronic medical conditions. If you have significant medical problems, even a low level of activity can be difficult for you. For instance, if you have had a stroke or if you have emphysema or lung disease, climbing a short flight of stairs may be the most exertion you can do.

Many people develop heart disease as they get older, and this can have a significant effect on mobility. If you have heart disease, even when you are resting and doing nothing, your heart may not be pumping as efficiently. Heart disease also may mean that when you get up and walk around your heart is not able keep up with your activity level. If this is the case, you may become fatigued even by simply walking around your house.

Improving Your Overall Conditioning

Even if you are not presently in good shape, no matter what your age or health problems, you can improve your level of fitness by following an exercise program. Exercise is the most important factor in determining how conditioned your heart and circulatory system can be. You are never too out of shape or too old to benefit from a training program! However, if you are over 40 you should consult your physician before starting a fitness program.

The main goal of any conditioning program is to increase the ability of the heart and muscles to do work. When you exercise in ways that makes your heart pump faster and harder, you improve your overall level of fitness. After you start an exercise program you should notice that it becomes easier to do things like climb stairs and walk at a fast pace.

How to Determine Your Exercise Intensity

With any exercise training program, the conditioning effect is accomplished by exercising hard enough to increase your heart rate. Studies have shown that to get a "conditioning" effect, you need to work at 60% of your maximum heart rate for 20 minutes three times a week. You may benefit from working at a higher intensity of exercise but be sure to check with your physician first.

The general formula used to determine your exercise heart rate is to subtract your age from 220 (this is your maximum heart rate) and then multiply that number by 60%. For example, if you are 75 years old, the formula would be:

$$220 - 75 = 145 \times .60 = 87.$$

So for you, about 85 to 90 beats per minute would be your exercise heart rate. This formula is only a guideline. More important than your heart rate is how you feel as you are exercising. You want to exercise with enough intensity to feel slightly fatigued with the workout.

Although for many people an appropriate conditioning program is determined by working at a specific heart rate, this is not true for all older adults. Certain medical conditions can affect your heart rate so that it does not increase much with exercise. Many blood pressure and heart medicines also have the effect of preventing your heart rate from speeding up.

Even if you can't rely on your heart rate to tell you the right level of exercise, you still can do conditioning exercises. Instead of working up to a certain heart rate, you can work up to a certain level of exertion. Research has shown that people can use how they feel very effectively, in place of determining their heart rate, to tell how hard to exercise. You should aim for a level of exertion that feels *fairly light* for you.

Tips for a Successful Conditioning Program

1. Before you start a new exercise program, check with your doctor to be sure that you don't have any medical problems that would make such exercises dangerous. Your physician can tell you if using heart rate to determine the intensity of exercise is appropriate for you or if you should simply base your exercise intensity on how hard the exercise feels to you.

An exercise test may be recommended before you start a new conditioning program. During an exercise test, your blood pressure and heart rate will be monitored while you ride a bicycle, walk a treadmill, or pedal with your arms. You will be evaluated to make sure you do not have any cardiac problems while you are doing the test.

2. Start slowly! Although you will be working up to a goal of 20 minutes of exercise at a time, this is not where you should start. If you are starting a new activity, you should begin with several short periods of exercise with breaks in between. For instance, you can start with two morning exercise periods of 3 to 5 minutes each with a rest in between and then two afternoon exercise periods for the same amount of time. This way you will get a total of 12 to 20 minutes of exercise a day.

You can gradually build up to doing two 10 minute exercise periods a day. From there, gradually increase your exercise tolerance until you can exercise 20 minutes at a time without a break.

3. To get the full conditioning effect, you should do your training program three to five times a week. You do not need to exercise every day. Giving yourself several days a week off from exercising will let your body rest and prevent you from overfatiguing any muscles.

4. It is very important to "warm-up" and "cool down" when exercising. Warm-up and cool-down periods are designed to stretch the muscles you are working. Keeping your muscles flexible helps prevent muscle injury or strain. Do warm-up stretches of your legs and back (see Chapter 5) for at least 5 minutes before starting your conditioning exercise program. At the end of your training activity, "cool-down" your muscles for another 5 minutes by doing the stretches over again.

5. Choose an exercise you enjoy. This will help you develop a program that you will want to stick with. For example, if you enjoy exercising with people, a group fitness class may suit your needs. If you enjoy peaceful time alone, a solitary walking program may work best for you. Don't be afraid to experiment a little. The first activity you pick may not be the best for you. If that's the case, try another.

6. Many people find they need some structure to continue with an exercise program. Doing exercises at about the same time every day is helpful. For example, walking before lunch every day or swimming first thing in the morning may provide you with an exercise routine that you can follow on a regular basis.

7. You need to be careful in extreme temperatures. If it is very cold, with the temperature below freezing, you should be cautious when exercising outdoors. Everyone has heard of people who have heart attacks while shoveling snow. When you exercise outdoors in cold weather, you may work harder than you realize. It is more difficult to judge your level of exertion because you are not as likely to feel warm or perspire. In general, when the temperature is into the mid to lower teens, it is wise to stay indoors to exercise.

It also is important to avoid strenuous activity outside in very hot weather. As you get older, you do not adapt as well in warm temperatures and you increase the risk of getting overheated. People have different tolerances for heat. If it feels too hot outside for you to be comfortable, exercise indoors. In general, if the temperature is over 90 degrees, exercise where there is air conditioning.

8. Know your limits in exercising! If you are following your pulse, slow down if your rate exceeds your exercise heart rate [(220 − age) × 0.6]. Whether or not you check your pulse, if the exertion starts to feel somewhat hard to you, slow down or stop. You do not need to overexert yourself to achieve a conditioning effect.

9. Most importantly, stop if you develop chest pain, nausea, or dizziness. Notify your doctor if you develop these symptoms while you are doing your conditioning program. If you begin to feel sick in any way, you should stop exercising and resume only when you feel well.

Specific Training Programs

There are many different kinds of conditioning activities. Walking, jogging, swimming, or bicycling all can improve your overall level of conditioning. A training program can be a very simple plan of walking for a certain amount of time or a certain distance several days a week. On the other hand, a training program can be complex and structured around using exercise equipment or attending a fitness center. Whatever program you choose, training needs to be done several times a week to achieve and maintain the benefits of conditioning. Listed below are specific activities which can help you improve your conditioning.

Group Fitness Programs

Many senior centers and YMCAs offer aerobic exercise classes that are structured for older adults. They include warm-up and cool-down periods. Exercise classes vary in intensity from easy to strenuous. Some classes provide conditioning exercises that can be done while sitting down. Chair exercises are ideal for older adults who have mobility problems. Ask the program staff members for complete details on types of exercises that are offered.

Bicycling

Bicycling is an excellent conditioning activity. Biking is a good outdoor exercise in the summer and is also a suitable winter activity using a stationary indoor bicycle. When biking a number of precautions should be taken:

1. Use a bike that fits you properly. The seat height should be adjusted so that your knees bend and straighten comfortably as the pedals are turned. When the pedal is at its lowest point, your knee should remain slightly bent.

2. Adjust the gears or set the resistance at a low enough level to avoid excessive force on your knees. You want to pedal at an intensity that feel fairly light to you.

3. Avoid steep hills that require you to pedal excessively hard.

4. Don't bike on rough terrain where you are at a risk of losing your balance and falling.

5. Wear a bicycle helmet if you are biking outside. If you are involved in a biking accident the risk of a serious head injury is greatly reduced by wearing a helmet. Just as you should never ride in a car without wearing a seat belt, you should never ride a bicycle without wearing a helmet.

Even if you have arthritis, you may be still be able to ride a bicycle. Just be sure to check with your doctor for guidance before starting a cycling program. Extra caution may be needed so you do not cause undue stress on your joints.

Swimming

Swimming can be done individually or through a group program. It is usually tolerated well by people with arthritis or other chronic medical problems. Swimming is appropriate for people who are relatively deconditioned as well as those who are highly trained. Water can be used either to give buoyancy and limit the amount of effort needed to exercise or as resistance to increase the amount of work you do.

Walking

For most people, walking is the easiest exercise to do. Even people with limited mobility often can do some walking to remain active. Walking certainly is the most practical form of exercise for most people. It also can be structured easily into a year-round conditioning program. In warm weather, many people prefer to walk outdoors. During the winter, indoor mall walking is a good alternative. If you enjoy group activities, some cities have mall-walking-clubs you can join.

Walking is adaptable to different levels of intensity. When you start a new walking program, remember to tailor it to your current level of fitness. Listed below are various levels for starting a walking fitness program along with hints to help you decide what level is right for you.

The goal in all the levels is to gradually increase your walking time and speed. You should walk at least 20 minutes 3 times a week at an intensity that causes you to reach your target heart rate or to feel an exertion level which is fairly light.

Level One

If you are somewhat out of shape, so that you do only occasional light housework or chores, this level is appropriate for you. If you have medical problems that impair your mobility, you also should start with this level. Begin by walking no more than 2 city blocks (about 1/10 mile) at a time, using a walking pace that feels natural to you. Try to do two walks a day. Slowly increase your walking speed and distance as you become more conditioned. Add 1/2 to 1 block every week, until you are walking for 20 minutes at a time.

Level Two

If you are somewhat more fit and regularly do house- or yard work, you can start by walking about 4 or 5 city blocks. Again, start at a pace that feels natural to you. Gradually build up the distance you walk, being sure to rest as needed. Also gradually increase the speed you walk so that you exert yourself enough to receive a conditioning effect from walking. You should feel you have gotten a fairly light workout by the end of the walk.

Level Three

If you can comfortably do heavy housework or yard work, you probably will be able to start with this level.

Begin walking about 1/2 mile at a pace that is slightly brisk for you. You can progress slowly over several weeks by increasing both the distance and speed with which you walk until you are walking for 20 to 30 minutes four to five times a week.

Summary

Keeping in good shape is essential as you get older. Being in good condition ensures that both your heart and muscles will continue to work efficiently. Regardless of how old you are, by following a fitness training program, you can increase your overall level of conditioning. This will allow you to be the most active and mobile that you can be.

Chapter 7

Dizziness and Unsteadiness

Dizziness and unsteadiness are common problems as people get older. Unfortunately, feelings of dizziness or unsteadiness can have a big impact on mobility. These feelings may cause you to have significant trouble with walking and often are a factor in falling.

What people mean when they say they are dizzy varies from person to person. To some people, it means feeling weak, faint, or lightheaded. To others, dizziness means vertigo, which is the feeling of the room spinning around. Unsteadiness also means different things to different people. It often refers to the feeling of simply having trouble keeping your equilibrium or balance.

Lightheadedness

What Is Lightheadedness?

There is no single medical definition for lightheadedness. However, most people have experienced the feeling. You probably recognize the sensation you feel when you stand up from a chair too fast or get up suddenly from a bent over position. You feel as if you could faint. This is also sometimes referred to as wooziness.

Lightheadedness does not occur only when you change positions. You can have feelings of lightheadedness that come on regardless of the position you are in. Although lightheaded or woozy feelings usually are temporary and go away very quickly, you can have feelings of lightheadedness that last for longer periods of time.

There are many causes of lightheadedness. Figuring out what to do about lightheadedness depends on what is causing it. Some of the causes and solutions are listed below.

Orthostatic Lightheadedness

"Orthostatic lightheadedness" is one of the most common types of lightheadedness. This refers to the feeling of faintness you sometimes get when you go from lying or sitting to standing very quickly. When you stand up from a chair or get up suddenly from crouching, stooping, or bending, your blood pressure may suddenly drop well below what it usually is and this can cause you to feel faint.

You do not need to have low blood pressure to feel lightheadedness when you change position from lying or sitting to standing. This type of problem with lightheadedness can develop even if your blood pressure usually is normal or even high. Regardless of what your blood pressure generally runs, if it drops significantly as you go from sitting to standing you may experience lightheadedness.

What You Can Do

If you have orthostatic lightheadedness, that is, lightheadedness that comes on when you stand up, there are certain things you can do to prevent yourself from falling or fainting.

1. When you first stand up, the best tactic is to hold onto something until you are certain you are not feeling lightheaded.

2. Also after kneeling or crouching, get up slowly, not all at once. When getting out of bed, instead of standing up immediately, sit on the edge of the bed for a minute or two first. This will give your blood pressure time to adjust so it does not drop as much when you stand up.

3. Another tip is to pump your ankles up and down several times before you stand up. This will help pump the blood from your feet and legs up toward your head.

4. Your doctor may recommend special support stockings to treat this type of lightheadedness. Elastic stockings help push the blood up from your legs toward your upper body and help keep your blood pressure from dropping too low as you change positions. The sections on dehydration and blood pressure medication in Chapter 10 give more information on what to do if you have this type of lightheadedness.

Causes of Orthostatic Lightheadedness

Some people have orthostatic lightheadedness all the time whenever they change positions. Other people experience this problem only rarely. A number of different medical problems can predispose you to having this type of lightheadedness. Some of the most common causes are discussed below.

Dehydration

You can develop lightheadedness with position changes if you have not been drinking the amount of water that you need. If you are dehydrated, you may not have a sufficient volume of water in your blood. As a result, your blood pressure can drop too low, and you may notice wooziness when you first stand up or start to walk.

As you get older, your thirst drive is not as strong so it is easy to get behind on the amount of fluids you need. In summer heat or when you are physically active, your need for fluids increases. This is when you are most prone to getting dehydrated.

What You Can Do

1. If you notice you are getting lightheaded with position changes, think about the amount of fluids you are drinking. Check page 147 ("Dehydration, What You Can Do") for specifics on how much fluid to drink in a day.

2. When you are physically active, such as when you are working around the house or exercising, remember that you need to increase the amount of liquids you drink.

3. Also in the summertime be aware of how much you are drinking. Particularly in the summer, if you develop feelings of faintness or lightheadedness when you change positions, you probably need to drink more fluids.

Illness

Another major cause of a blood pressure drop when you change position is illness. For instance, everyone is familiar with getting the flu and feeling lightheaded. Colds, infections, and diarrhea all can cause you to feel weak and faint, especially when you first stand up.

What You Can Do. If your lightheadedness is related to a flu or another illness, as with dehydration, it is important to drink plenty of fluids. Soups and broths, which tend to be salty, are especially good for meeting your fluid requirements because they contain sodium. When you are dehydrated, you often are depleted of sodium.

CAUTION: For some people, consuming salty beverages and foods can lead to excess water retention and swelling in the legs or around the ankles. If you have a problem with ankle swelling, check with your physician before you drink a lot of salty liquids.

Medications

Many different blood pressure medications can cause your blood pressure to temporarily drop too low when you are getting up from a chair or from lying down. These medicines can lead to a feeling of lightheadedness as you change positions.

Besides blood pressure medications, other types of drugs also can cause lightheadedness with position changes. Drugs used to treat depression commonly have lightheadedness as a side effect. Some over-the-counter cold medicines and anti-allergy preparations also can cause lightheaded feelings as you stand up.

What You Can Do. If you begin to have lightheadedness that comes on when you change positions, and the problem does not go away in a few days, check with your doctor. It may be that one of your medications is contributing to the problem. Your doctor may substitute another similar type of drug that does not have the same degree of side effects as the one you are taking. Be sure to tell your doctor about any nonprescription medicines you are taking. They also can be contributing to your lightheadedness.

Other Types of Lightheadedness

You may have lightheadedness that occurs regardless of what position you are in and even if you have not just changed positions. You may feel woozy even when you are lying down. This type of lightheadedness is not necessarily related to a drop in blood pressure. It can be caused by a number of different problems. Hunger and hyperventilation are two common causes.

Hunger

Hunger can cause a feeling of weakness and lightheadedness. If you are working hard and miss a regularly scheduled meal, you may feel a little lightheaded. It is very rare, however, for this type of problem to lead to fainting.

What You Can Do

1. If you tend to develop lightheadedness when you are very hungry, try to keep a light snack with you at all times. Avoid high sugar snacks, however, because this type of meal is digested quickly and can lead to having the same lightheaded feelings again in another hour or two. The best snacks are a mixture of complex sugars and proteins, a sandwich, for example, or fruits and nuts together.

2. Eating regularly scheduled meals can help you avoid lightheadedness resulting from getting too hungry. Again, well balanced meals that include complex sugars and proteins work better than meals of high sugar foods.

Hyperventilation

Breathing too fast, which is called "hyperventilation," can cause you to feel lightheaded. Hyperventilating is not something people normally do. However, it can happen if you feel anxious. Even if you are not aware of it, whenever you are nervous or anxious, you naturally speed up your breathing. After about a minute of rapid breathing you can become quite lightheaded and may feel faint.

What You Can Do. If you are feeling anxious or nervous and then get lightheaded, check to see if you are breathing too rapidly. How do you do this? A person normally breathes 12 to 16 times per minute. If you notice that you are breathing very rapidly, for instance over 20 times a minute, try slowing your breathing down by exhaling very slowly and pausing before taking your next breath. If your feeling of faintness is related to hyperventilation, as your breathing slows down you immediately will notice that you feel much better.

Vertigo

What is Vertigo?

Vertigo is a distinct type of dizziness. It is the feeling that things are moving while you are standing still or that you are spinning or moving while the rest of the world is standing still.

Vertigo is a specific medical condition caused by a problem with the inner ear or with the nerves that go from the inner ear to the brain. The inner ear contains the center that detects motion whenever your head moves. When your inner ear system is working properly, when you turn your head you are aware that only your head is moving. The rest of the your body and the environment around you are still.

When this system is not working properly, every time you turn your head you may feel like your entire body is moving. You may feel as if you are on a boat or a swing and having motion sickness. Or when you turn your head, you may feel that you are still, but everything is rotating or spinning around you. Along with vertigo you may have nausea and vomiting.

What Causes Vertigo?

Viral Infections

Some types of viral infections can cause attacks of vertigo. If you have one of these viral infections, any movement can bring on the feeling of spinning. Because the symptoms are so severe, and because any head movement can bring them on, vertigo resulting from such a viral infection is very disabling. However, it usually is not permanent. It typically lasts only several days to a week, and then resolves completely.

What You Can Do

1. Because the feeling of vertigo often is so severe as to make it difficult to walk, bed rest usually is required. If you remain still, without turning your head, the feelings of vertigo are least noticeable.

2. If you develop severe vertigo, be sure to notify your doctor so you can be examined to determine if a viral infection is causing the problem.

Although there is no treatment specifically for these viral infections, the severity of the symptoms may be improved by taking medications that relieve motion sickness.

Benign Positional Vertigo

A common cause of a spinning sensation is benign positional vertigo, which occurs in 10 to 20% of all people who report symptoms of dizziness. The cause is not known, but it is characterized by a sensation of spinning that comes on with head turning and lasts only a few seconds to several minutes. Benign positional vertigo also can occur when you go from lying to sitting or from sitting to lying. This type of vertigo is not as severe as the vertigo caused by viral infections. It usually is more annoying than disabling.

What You Can Do

1. If you have benign positional vertigo, it is important to remember to be extra careful whenever you change positions or turn your head. This is when you will have the symptoms and be most likely to lose your balance.

2. If the vertigo is severe and significantly interferes with your balance and your ability to get around, notify your doctor. Your physician can prescribe medication to relieve the spinning sensation.

3. After examining you to make sure of the cause of your dizziness, your doctor may also prescribe head movement exercises. These exercises are designed to build up your tolerance for head turning and rotation so that you are not as likely to get symptoms.

Meniere's Disease

Meniere's disease can cause a spinning type of dizziness. This disease typically begins when people are in their forties or fifties. It is characterized by hearing loss, ringing in the ears, and episodic dizziness which can last from minutes to hours. The course of Meniere's disease is noted for having remissions and relapses. You may have a flare up of dizziness, and then it may get better on its own. Although this is not a very common disease, for people who have it, their ability to get around can be significantly impaired.

What You Can Do

1. Just like with other causes of vertigo, the first thing to do is see your physician. Before beginning any treatment you need to find out what is causing your dizziness.

2. As with other causes of vertigo, it helps to be extra careful with head movement and position changes because this is what brings on the spinning sensations. This includes looking up and looking down, as well as turning the head from side to side.

3. It is also important for you to remember to keep good lighting in the house at all times. Light maximizes your vision, and this will help you compensate for balance problems. Take extra caution when walking in dim light because these are times when you may have particular trouble with your balance.

Medications

Certain types of drugs can cause damage to the inner ear and lead to a spinning type of dizziness. If you take a lot of aspirin, for example, you may develop dizziness or inner ear damage. Also certain diuretics or water pills if taken in large doses can cause inner ear problems.

What You Can Do. If you develop a new spinning sensation, or a sensation of things moving, check with your physician. Be sure to tell your doctor all of the medications you are taking. Your doctor may recommend that you cut back or stop taking any medicines that could be causing or worsening the problem.

Unsteadiness

What Is Unsteadiness?

Unsteadiness is the feeling of not having good balance. You can feel unsteady without actually feeling dizzy. You may simply feel that you cannot keep your balance when you walk or move. Feelings of unsteadiness often are associated with problems walking. If you are unsteady, you may walk with uneven or staggering steps. On the other hand, you can feel unsteady but still walk fairly normally.

What Causes Unsteadiness?

Feelings of unsteadiness can indicate a problem in the brain or be a side effect of drugs acting on the brain, a problem with the inner ear, or a problem with the nerves that carry messages from the feet and legs to the brain.

Various brain disorders can cause feelings of unsteadiness or problems in walking. These include certain types of infections, tumors, and strokes. Many drugs also can affect the parts of the brain that control walking and cause feelings of unsteadiness. Sleeping medications, in particular, can cause this problem. Alcohol is another drug that causes unsteadiness, and it can lead to a staggering pattern of walking. Alcohol affects the areas of the brain that control coordination and smoothness of movement.

Problems in the inner ear sometimes also cause feelings of unsteadiness. Sometimes this type of unsteadiness may worsen when you turn your head. This is because your inner ear helps stabilize you when you turn your head. If your inner ear is not functioning properly, when your head moves, you lose your sense of stability.

If the nerves in the spinal cord or legs are damaged, which can happen in a number of diseases, you also may feel unsteady. Intact nerves are essential to relay sensations from the feet and legs to the brain. Vitamin deficiencies, chronic alcohol abuse, and diabetes, as well as other diseases, all may lead to damage in the nerves in the spinal cord or legs.

What You Can Do. If you are unsteady, the first thing to do is see your doctor to determine your diagnosis. Continuing to walk as much as possible is essential. There are a number of very important and relatively simple things you can do to make your walking safer.

1. See a physical therapist. A physical therapist can provide balance training and help you improve your walking to some extent, even if complete recovery of a normal walking pattern is not possible. Various types of canes and walkers frequently are helpful in increasing stability. You should be assessed by a physical therapist to see which, if any, walking aid is best for you. Chapter 13 describes various types of assistive devices in more detail.

2. Make sure you have supervision if you need it. Having someone guide your walking sometimes is the best solution for safety. If you need hands-on assistance to walk safely, you may be advised to wear a gait belt. This is a wide belt worn around the waist. The person who is assisting you holds onto the belt while you are walking. Before using a gait belt, you should get instructions from a physical therapist or other person who has been specially trained in how to use the belt properly.

3. Pay attention to your footwear. To be as safe as possible when you walk, you need to wear appropriate footwear. Check your shoes and slippers to make sure they do not have slippery soles. Remember that walking in stocking feet is always risky, especially if you are already unsteady. For additional information on footwear, see Chapter 12.

4. Be extra cautious when you are tired or ill. If you have an unsteady gait, for whatever reason, it is extremely important for you to be aware of factors that can make your unsteadiness worse. A minor illness such as a cold can make walking more difficult. Fatigue also can be a big problem. If you are tired from physical exertion or from the day's activities, you may notice that your walking becomes more unsteady. Getting enough sleep and taking frequent short rests during the day can prevent deterioration toward the end of the day.

5. Be aware of drug side effects. If you have a problem with unsteadiness, it is very important to remember that you may be more susceptible to the side effects of certain drugs such as sleeping pills and alcohol. Sleeping pills can cause your walking to become more unsteady and even a small drink of alcohol may have an exaggerated effect on your mobility and safety. Seizure drugs are another type of medication that often cause unsteadiness or difficulty in walking.

If you have problems with unsteadiness, check with your doctor whenever you start a new nonprescription drug or change dosages of a drug you are already taking. Because virtually any medicine can affect mobility, remember to always take the lowest possible dose that you can.

Summary

If you have lightheadedness, vertigo, or unsteadiness, your mobility most likely will be limited to some extent. However, there are a number of things you can do to improve both your walking and your confidence in getting around safely. Being more careful whenever you move or change positions is one of the keys to making your activities safe. By taking extra caution with your movements and getting the proper medical treatment, you can keep yourself as active as possible!

Chapter 8

Arthritis

Arthritis is a painful, chronic condition that affects millions of older Americans. There are many different types of arthritis, but what they all have in common is pain and stiffness of the joints. Almost half of all people over the age of 65 have some sort of problem with arthritis. It is one of the leading causes of disability for older adults and a major cause of impaired mobility.

What is Arthritis?

Some people refer to arthritis as "rheumatism." Regardless of the name, it is a chronic, disabling disease of the joints. Although arthritis often is thought of as an inevitable part of growing old, it is not, in fact, a normal part of aging.

By far, the majority of people with arthritis have osteoarthritis, which also is known as degenerative joint disease. A much smaller number of people have rheumatoid arthritis, which is a very different disease.

What is Rheumatoid Arthritis?

Rheumatoid arthritis affects many organs in the body in addition to the joints. Although rheumatoid arthritis usually starts during young adulthood, it can start at any age, even during childhood. In this disease, the immune system turns against the body's own tissues. This immune response is most noticeable in the joints, where chronic inflammation occurs.

Treatment of Rheumatoid Arthritis

If you have rheumatoid arthritis, you should be under the care of a physician. Drugs that suppress the body's immune response usually are helpful in controlling the disease. Because joint involvement in rheumatoid arthritis may be severe, you should consult your physician before starting an exercise program. Some of the suggestions discussed in this chapter may help you cope with mobility problems related to rheumatoid arthritis.

What is Osteoarthritis?

Osteoarthritis involves only the joints, not other organs of the body. It is like rheumatoid arthritis in that joint inflammation sometimes develops. However, osteoarthritis differs from rheumatoid arthritis in that it is not caused by a problem in the immune system itself.

How Does Osteoarthritis Develop?

Osteoarthritis begins when joint cartilage starts to break down. Cartilage provides a smooth rubbery padding between your bones. When the cartilage wears down from osteoarthritis, you lose this smooth surface, and the joint covering becomes pitted and irregular. This can lead to pain and stiffness. Sometimes inflammation occurs in response to the wearing down of cartilage, and as a result the joints may swell.

As the disease progresses, more and more cartilage wears down, allowing the bones on both sides of the joint to come into direct contact with each other. If this happens in the hip or knee joints, when the cartilage disappears, the bones actually may grind against each other as you walk. This usually produces such a significant amount of pain that you may try to avoid walking as much as possible.

Along with the destruction of cartilage, the bones around the involved joint tend to overgrow. New bone tissue is formed around the joint (see the illustration below). For example, with knee osteoarthritis, the ends of the calf and thigh bones develop excessive bone and grow toward each other. As a result the distance between the two bones gets shorter and the knee joint may become enlarged and deformed.

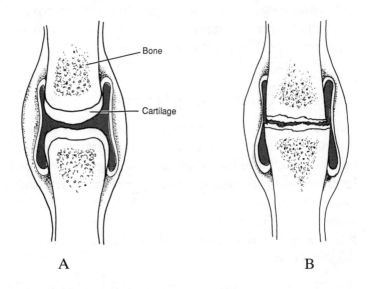

A. Normal joint. B. Joint with osteoarthritis.

What Joints Are Involved in Osteoarthritis?

Any joint can develop osteoarthritis. The hands frequently are affected, and the knee and hip also commonly are involved. Osteoarthritis quite often involves the joints of the back and neck as well.

Do Men and Women Get Osteoarthritis the Same Way?

Women and men tend to be affected differently by this disease. Men are more likely to get osteoarthritis in the spine and hips. Women are more likely to develop it in the hands, knees, ankles, and feet. Although women and men tend to have slightly different patterns of joint involvement, any person, regardless of gender, can develop osteoarthritis in any joint.

What Causes Osteoarthritis?

No one has been able to pinpoint the exact cause of osteoarthritis. It is not primarily a hereditary disease, and old age alone is not enough to cause it. Osteoarthritis tends to occur in the presence of a number of different factors. Two of the most important and most common factors are obesity and mechanical stress on the joint. The presence of either of these factors makes it more likely that a person will develop arthritis.

1. Obesity. Being overweight may contribute to osteoarthritis because it increases the mechanical wear and tear on the joints. The knees are especially prone to developing arthritis when obesity is present.

2. Mechanical Stress. Exercise does not cause arthritis, but it can contribute to more wear and tear on a joint if injury is already present. If mechanical stress from strenuous exercise is repeatedly superimposed on a previously injured joint, the cartilage can become inflamed, and permanent damage can occur. Over time, this mechanical stress may lead to arthritis.

How is Osteoarthritis Diagnosed?

The most important symptom of arthritis is pain. The pain of osteoarthritis typically increases with movement of the joint and improves with rest. As the disease progresses, however, the pain may be present even when the joint is not moving. Night pain may occur and can interfere with sleeping.

The other major symptom of osteoarthritis is stiffness in the affected joint. Sometimes, but not usually, fluid collects in the joint and causes swelling. Even with swelling and pain, however, it is very unusual to see any redness in a joint with osteoarthritis.

How Does Osteoarthritis Limit People?

The pain associated with arthritis often leads to limitations in mobility and physical activity. People who experience arthritis pain may guard their joints in an attempt to prevent discomfort without even realizing they are doing so. For example, they may cut down on the amount of walking they do or change their walking pattern to protect the involved joint. People also may start consciously protecting a painful joint. For example, they may avoid going up and down stairs because of arthritis in their hips or knees.

In addition to having pain, some people with arthritis have joints that unexpectedly lock or buckle because of loose pieces of cartilage. If this happens while a person is walking, a fall can result. People may find they limit their walking out of fear that this will happen.

Unfortunately, limiting activity because of pain or fear of falling is not the best treatment for the disease. Muscles get weaker from lack of use and then they do not protect the joint as well. Also, lack of use causes the joints to stiffen. Stiffness will make the pain worse and lead to loss of joint flexibility. A progressive loss of joint range of motion then leads to further loss of mobility.

As people lose mobility, they also lose cardiovascular conditioning. They gradually decrease their tolerance for exercise. As a result, they will find it harder to continue such basic activities as going up stairs or walking up a ramp. For all of these reasons, to maintain muscle strength, keep joints flexible, and maintain cardiovascular conditioning, it is best to keep as active as possible.

How is Osteoarthritis Treated?

One of the primary goals of treatment of osteoarthritis is pain relief. Although some decrease in pain can be achieved, complete relief of pain is not always possible. Another primary goal of treatment is improvement in function and mobility. Inherent in improving function is an increase in flexibility and strength.

Treatment of osteoarthritis generally is directed toward measures to help patients cope with the disease. Mainstays of living with arthritis are continuing physical activities that can help arthritis, avoiding physical activities that worsen the disease, losing weight if appropriate, and following physician guidance regarding pain-relieving medications. There also are surgical procedures that can increase mobility when other measures are not successful.

Physical Activities to Help Arthritis

It is a common misconception that strengthening exercises should be avoided with arthritis. Many people fear that an active physical fitness program will aggravate the disease. In fact, physical activity is an essential part of the treatment for restoring and maintaining mobility for people who have osteoarthritis.

A daily exercise program designed to keep the affected joints limber is a cornerstone of treatment for arthritis. Exercise is useful for increasing range of motion and strengthening the muscles around the joint, as well as for improving overall conditioning. Stretching and strengthening are the two main types of exercise you should do for arthritis. Hints on both of these types of exercise are described below.

Stretching Exercises

Specific stretching exercises are described in Chapter 5. Stretching activities are very helpful for keeping all your joints mobile. They are especially important for joints that have arthritis, because these joints are particularly susceptible to stiffening. If done properly, these exercises should not increase arthritis pain.

Tips for Following a Stretching Program

1. Stretching exercises should be done in a relaxed, nonstressful position. The best position for doing leg stretches is sitting or lying down. Arm stretches can be done lying, sitting, or standing. Trunk and neck exercises are best done sitting or standing.

2. The key to doing stretching exercises properly is to do them slowly, gently, and smoothly. Stretch the joints as much as you can without exacerbating pain. Initially, you should start by doing just a few exercises at a time. As you become more limber, you can increase the number of repetitions and the variety of stretching exercises you do each day.

3. If you develop new or increased joint pain after starting a flexibility exercise program, you should consult your physician or a physical therapist. Individualized instruction in a stretching program designed specifically for you may be necessary.

4. Chapter 5 presents a number of stretching exercises that can help you start your flexibility program. Remember to choose exercises that stretch the joints that have arthritis.

Strengthening Exercises

Chapter 3 gives some good strengthening exercises that you may try. Strengthening the muscles around the affected joints is an important part of your treatment plan. Keeping the muscles strong will help protect your joints from added strain. For instance, if your thigh muscles are strong, when you get up from a chair, the muscles can easily generate the force needed for you to get up. As a result your legs will be more likely to remain in good alignment and less stress will be placed on your knee joints.

Tips for Following a Strengthening Program

1. The key to doing strengthening exercises is to do them in the right way. Make your motions slow and smooth, and stop if you start to feel pain.

2. When you begin your strengthening program, start by doing only a few exercises at one time. The first few times you exercise a muscle you haven't worked before, you need to be cautious not to overdo the activity. If inflammation related to a new activity occurs, it may take several hours, or even until the next day, before pain or soreness is felt. Therefore, because you cannot anticipate how your muscles and joints will react to a new strengthening program, you should start with a minimum of activity and gradually build up.

3. You only need to do strengthening exercises every other day to get benefit from them. By not exercising every day you also will give your muscles a chance to rest between workouts.

4. Remember, if any exercise leads to pain, you should stop and start again slowly with smooth movements after the pain and soreness have resolved.

Other Activities to Help Arthritis

It is fine to do smooth, repetitive exercises such as swimming, biking, or walking as long as there is no jerking or jarring of the involved joints and the exercise does not aggravate pain. In fact, studies have shown that a regular walking program can actually help decrease arthritis pain! However, it is best to avoid activities like jogging or jumping-type aerobics because these activities can put undue strain on your joints.

It is important to remember to pace yourself when exercising or doing any activities such as housework or gardening that involve arthritic joints. Pacing means to rest between exercises or activities so you do not overdo and aggravate pain. Finally, if you have joints that sometimes lock or buckle, then, whatever your activity, you need to use extra caution to avoid a fall.

Physical Activities to Avoid (And How to Get Around Them)

Being aware of what worsens your osteoarthritis symptoms and modifying your daily activities to avoid pain as much as possible, while still remaining mobile, is a very important goal. This section describes ways you can change these physical activities to decrease joint pain and improve your level of functioning.

Carrying and Lifting Things

Some weight-bearing activities may be too stressful for a joint with arthritis and should be avoided. For example, carrying a heavy bag of groceries up a flight of stairs will aggravate a painful hip or knee. Lifting heavy objects, in general, may put too much force on an arthritic joint.

For the most part, however, it is okay to lift or carry light-weight objects. How you carry them, though, will make a difference. If you have hip arthritis and need to carry an item, such as a purse or a package, it is preferable to carry it on the side of the involved joint. If your right hip is arthritic, it would be better for that joint to carry your purse in your right hand or over your right shoulder. The reason to put the weight on the same side as the arthritic joint is that this allows the muscles around that joint to work more efficiently. When the muscles work more effectively, there is less stress on the joint itself.

Bending and Squatting

As a general rule, if you have osteoarthritis bending and squatting should be avoided because they put excess strain on the knees and hips. Usually it is difficult for people with hip or knee arthritis to squat. However, sometimes people do not realize that when they bend down to reach bottom cupboards or the closet floor, they are actually doing a deep knee bend. It is better for your joints if you rearrange cupboards and closets so that you do not need to bend or squat to reach frequently used items.

Changing Positions

Maintaining any one position for too long should be avoided because it will increase joint stiffness. If you have knee arthritis, it is helpful to stretch your legs frequently when you are sitting. While standing, it is best to shift your weight from side to side and avoid standing with most of your weight on one leg. Changing positions frequently will help keep your joints as flexible as possible.

Going Up and Down Stairs

In general, if an activity causes more pain in a joint, it should be avoided. For example, some people experience increased pain when walking up or down stairs. If this is the case, negotiating stairs should be avoided when possible. Use an elevator, escalator or ramp if one is available. If steps are difficult for a person who has an upstairs bedroom, it may be best to move the bedroom downstairs.

Tips for Negotiating Stairs. If you need to go up and down stairs or curbs, a number of tips can help.

1. When going up stairs, lead with the leg that has the least problem with arthritis. Place your strongest leg on the step first, then follow with your arthritic leg. Place both feet on each step, instead of walking step over step.

2. To descend stairs or a curb, place your arthritic leg down first, then follow with your noninvolved leg. These techniques for negotiating stairs put the least amount of strain on the arthritic joints.

3. Using a hand railing to help you go up and down stairs also is very helpful. Having a railing on both sides of a stairway is ideal because if the stairway is narrow enough you can hold onto a rail with both hands. If the stairway is wide or if you are carrying something, holding onto the railing on your strong side should make you feel the most secure.

Managing Housework and Gardening

The bending and kneeling involved in doing housework can increase joint pain from arthritis. If doing household chores causes more pain, you may need assistance with these activities. Assistance can range from hiring someone for help with chores, to accepting offers of help from a neighbor, friend, or relative. Modified cleaning devices that decrease the need for bending also are available. These include reachers and long-handled dustpans. Electric brooms are lightweight, smooth-floor vacuums that take the place of a broom and dustpan altogether.

Gardening also is an activity that may worsen arthritis symptoms. Planting a garden on an elevated plot eliminates the need to bend, squat, and kneel. Alternatively, it can be helpful to sit on a low, wheeled stool while you work in the garden.

Other Treatments for Arthritis

A variety of other treatments also can help decrease pain and improve your mobility if you have arthritis. Often a combination of these treatments is used either together or at different times.

Massage, Whirlpool, Heat, and Liniments

Massage and whirlpool baths may help decrease the muscle spasms that sometimes accompany painful arthritis. Moist heat also can be helpful. It is easy to make a hot, moist compress by wrapping a damp towel around a plastic-lined heating pad. This should be applied to a joint only for short periods of time, and the skin should be checked frequently to make sure it is not getting too hot. Liniments such as Ben-Gay® and Aspercreme® frequently are used in the treatment of arthritis. The massaging action of applying the ointment may be part of the reason why these work. The massage also acts as a counterirritant. It creates a sensation which the nerves perceive of as very strong. The strength of the sensation blocks some of the feeling of pain.

Splints

When there is a painful flare-up of an arthritic joint, rest of the involved joint is important. Splints immobilize a joint and allow it to rest (see illustration on the next page). Your physician may prescribe a splint for a painful joint. As soon as the pain subsides, however, you need to move the joint again. If you do not get the joint moving as soon as possible, you will lose both flexibility and strength. Therefore, it is important to remove a splint as soon as your doctor or therapist says it's okay.

Braces

Once you are moving a joint again, you may still need to support it. A brace stabilizes a joint while still allowing it to move. Braces most commonly are used on the lower extremities with knee or ankle arthritis. With knee arthritis there is sometimes an associated problem of loose ligaments which can worsen the disease process. A knee brace may help stabilize the joint if the ligaments are loose (see the illustration below). The extra stabilization a brace provides often helps reduce pain and prevent further joint injury. Mobility also may be improved when you use a brace because it provides extra support for the joint and allows you to continue walking.

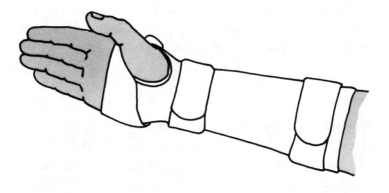

Wrist splint.

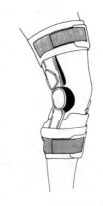

Knee brace.

Canes

With progression of arthritis, walking can become more painful. As you walk, you shift your weight from one foot to another. If you have hip or knee arthritis, as you shift your weight to the side of the affected joint, you may notice pain in that area. Fortunately, you can spare your affected hip or knee by using a cane. The cane will help redistribute your weight off the involved joint. To be effective, of course, a cane needs to be used correctly. Chapter 13 describes how to choose a cane and use it to your advantage.

Weight Loss

One of the most important, but often overlooked, treatments for arthritis is weight loss if obesity is a factor. Regardless of the length of time arthritis has been present, or the severity of symptoms, weight loss can be important in halting progression of the disease and decreasing pain.

Joint Injections

Sometimes a physician will inject an arthritic joint with an anti-inflammatory drug. This treatment usually is used when the main symptoms are confined to a single joint and fluid is present. It is unclear how many injections can safely be given in any one joint. Therefore, injections tend to be given only after other measures have been tried.

Surgery

Total joint replacement is the most commonly performed type of surgery for severe arthritis. Hips and knees are the most common sites for joint replacement surgery. These surgeries are not without risk of complications, but they may provide long-lasting pain relief and increased mobility. The main benefit of surgery is relief of pain. Joint replacements also can increase flexibility. You may find, for instance, that after a total knee replacement that you can fully extend your knee, whereas you were unable to fully straighten it before surgery.

If you have joint replacement surgery, you will begin rehabilitation training almost immediately after the operation. Although your hospitalization will last only a short time, your rehabilitation training will continue for several months. Strengthening and flexibility exercises will be started under the supervision of a physical therapist. The surgery itself is only a part of the treatment of joint replacement for osteoarthritis. Conscientiously following a prescribed exercise program after the surgery is a vital part of regaining your mobility.

Medications for Arthritis

Two main types of pain-relieving medications are commonly used to treat arthritis. The first, acetaminophen, or Tylenol®, helps relieve pain from chronic arthritis and has very few side effects. The second is a family of medications known as nonsteroidal anti-inflammatory drugs (NSAIDs). This class of drugs includes aspirin and ibuprofen which are nonprescription generic drugs and several prescription medications. Basically, all of the non-steroidal anti-inflammatory drugs work by reducing the inflammation which may be present in the joint. Unfortunately, although nonsteroidal anti-inflammatory drugs often are effective for relieving pain, they have many side effects, some of which may be life-threatening.

There is no good evidence that any one particular type of nonsteroidal anti-inflammatory drug is better than another. Some people will do better with one drug than another, but there is no way to predict which drug will work best ahead of time. Therefore, often it is a matter of trial and error to find the medication that works best for you.

An important thing to remember is that, when you are older, you most likely will not need as high a dose to get pain relief as a younger person. In general, the higher the dose you take, the more likely you are to get side effects. It is always recommended to start with the lowest suggested dose and then gradually increase it as needed. Before using any of the nonsteroidal anti-inflammatory drugs, even the nonprescription preparations, you should check with your physician. You also should consult your physician before making any change in dosage.

Side Effects of Nonsteroidal Anti-inflammatory Drugs

1. Irritation of the lining of the stomach

2. Stomach ulcer or bleeding from the stomach

3. Kidney damage

4. Fluid retention or swelling

If you notice black stools or significant swelling in your legs, you should stop taking the medication and call your doctor promptly.

In summary, medications can help relieve arthritis pain. It is probably safest to start with acetaminophen or Tylenol®; it may be all you need. If acetaminophen does not provide pain relief, after consultation with your doctor, you may be advised to try a nonsteroidal anti-inflammatory drug. A nonsteroidal anti-inflammatory drug may be quite helpful, but you need to be aware of all the side effects.

Summary

Arthritis is a major cause of difficulty with mobility in older adults. However, a variety of treatments can be used to improve, if not eliminate, the pain and loss of function that can occur because of arthritis. By following the guidelines provided on the various treatments for arthritis, you will be able to remain as active as possible.

Chapter 9

Osteoporosis

What is Osteoporosis?

Osteoporosis is a gradual loss of bone tissue that results in the bones becoming thin and fragile. It is a very common condition as people grow older. Half of all women and a third of all men will have osteoporosis by the age of 70.

Osteoporosis is a process that begins during young adulthood. From age 35 on everyone begins to lose some bone strength. Bone is continually being formed, but at the same time old bone is being removed. Early in life more bone is formed than destroyed, and this results in an increased amount of bone.

However, during and after middle age, slightly more bone is removed than is formed. As a result of this imbalance, the quantity of bone gradually decreases so that by age 65 or 70 a significant amount of bone can be lost. When the loss of bone becomes significant enough to be seen by special types of x-rays, or when fractures occur with minimal stress to the bone, the diagnosis of osteoporosis is made.

Osteoporosis and Fractures

Osteoporosis in and of it itself does not cause pain or problems with mobility. What it does do is increase the risk of fractures. As you lose bone, the bone that remains becomes weaker and weaker, and it takes less stress to cause it to break.

Fractures related to osteoporosis are common. By the age of 70 one out of four women will develop a fracture related to this disease. Men are not exempt from osteo-porotic fractures; however, fractures tend to occur later in life. Fractures of the vertebrae (back bones), wrist, and hip are the most common although other bones may break as well. All of these types of fractures are more common in women than in men until people reach the age of 80 when fracture rates in men and women become similar.

Compression Fractures

A compression fracture is a specific kind of fracture that occurs in the bones of the back. In this type of fracture, the bone crumbles and loses height. This happens asym-metrically, so that more crumbling occurs in the front than in the back of the bone. As the bone collapses in front, the spine curves forward. When many of the verte-brae in the back have compression fractures, the classic posture of a very rounded upper back often develops. This curved-forward posture is called kyphosis (see the illustration on the next page).

Compression fractures can occur with very little trauma. Sometimes they can result from something as simple as carrying a heavy object or missing a step and stumbling.

Do Compression Fractures Hurt?

Some compression fractures are not at all painful and occur without people being aware of them. At other times, however, they can be quite painful. Often the pain feels like a muscle strain, and muscle spasms frequently are present when a compression fracture occurs. Sometimes the pain is mild enough so that you can treat it on your own

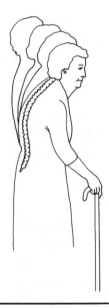

Kyphosis.

without seeing your doctor. At other times, the pain of compression fractures can be severe enough to require a doctor's attention. Unfortunately, with advanced osteoporosis, you can develop chronic back pain because of the presence of multiple compression fractures.

How Are Compression Fractures Treated?

Because there is no cure for compression fractures, treatment is aimed at relieving pain. Usually the pain associated with any one vertebrae fracture lasts 6 to 8 weeks. Bed rest may be helpful for the first several days following a compression fracture. However, it is important to keep bed rest to a minimum because it can lead to loss of strength, endurance, and flexibility.

A corset or a rigid brace may provide some pain relief. These devices support the abdominal muscles and help maintain an erect posture. Use of a back support may allow someone with a compression fracture to get out of bed sooner and regain mobility faster. However, there is a disadvantage to using corsets and braces. Muscle weakness can occur with prolonged use of these supports, and this can impair your mobility. As a result, corsets and braces should be used for the least amount of time possible.

How Do Compression Fractures Impair Mobility?

Compression fractures can limit your mobility in two major ways. First, as vertebrae collapse, your back becomes less flexible and more rounded. Kyphosis, or an excessively rounded upper back, will restrict your ability to straighten, bend, and turn. Walking may become slower and somewhat painful as a result of the back's limited movement. Exercising may be more difficult after a compression fracture and your back muscles may lose strength as your posture becomes more curved.

The second way compression fractures can limit your mobility is through pain. If you have back pain due to compression fractures, any activity that involves movement of the back may exacerbate pain. Simple tasks such as bending to make a bed or reaching overhead to the cupboards can be extraordinarily difficult for you if you have compression fractures.

Using Good Posture to Protect Against Compression Fractures

Lifting objects properly is essential to prevent undue pressure on the vertebrae. With any work that involves the back, be it pushing, pulling, bending, lifting, or reaching, you should remember to maintain good back alignment. The key to protecting your back when lifting is to keep your back straight at all times.

When lifting or moving anything, start by getting close to the object. Then bend at the hips and knees, so that your leg muscles, not your back, do the work. Your back should be straight when you start lifting the object. Tighten your abdominal muscles as you stand up to lift the weight. Strong stomach muscles act as a "brace" to keep your back stable (see the illustration below).

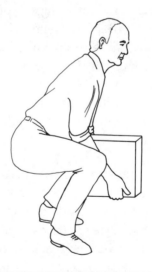

Technique for lifting.

Risk Factors for Osteoporosis

The most important risk factor for osteoporosis is age. The older you get, the more likely you are to have osteoporosis. Being female is the other major risk factor. Women get osteoporosis more than twice as often as men. Estrogen helps maintain bone strength. As women produce less estrogen after menopause, their bones become weaker and the risk of osteoporosis increases.

Other risk factors for developing osteoporosis include having a small body frame, having a parent or sibling with osteoporosis, and being of white or oriental race. You do not really have any control over these risk factors. However, there are other risk factors that you can modify. These include a sedentary lifestyle, low calcium and Vitamin D intake, smoking, and excessive use of alcohol. It is important to remember that these risk factors matter throughout your life, even if you already have osteoporosis.

Diagnosis

Advanced osteoporosis is easy to detect on plain x-rays. The appearance of the bones is less dense, and fractures in the spine or other bones of the body are easily visible. Of course, ideally osteoporosis should be detected before fractures occur. This is particularly true for people who are at high risk for developing the disease. If early detection was possible, people could start treatment before fractures occur. Unfortunately, early osteoporosis cannot be detected by plain x-rays. One third of the bone needs to be lost before the disease will be visible on regular x-rays of the spine. Recently, new types of x-ray-like machines have been developed that can detect osteoporosis at earlier stages in the wrist, spine, or hip. Your doctor can determine whether this special testing would be beneficial for you.

Preventative Treatment

The best treatment for osteoporosis is prevention! Although bone loss starts in middle age, the first 30 years of your life are important in determining how much total bone mass you have. No matter what your age, there are things you can do to help reduce the amount of bone loss that occurs. These preventative measures are exercise and a diet adequate in calcium and vitamin D.

Exercise and Physical Activity

Exercise and physical activity play a major role in increasing bone density when you are young. Both also are essential for maintaining bone mass as you age. For people who have already developed osteoporosis, exercise can help prevent further bone loss.

Specific Types of Exercises

Upright, weight-bearing activities are the most useful for increasing bone formation. The degree of bone formation is directly related to the amount of weight and stress placed on your bones. Weight-bearing activities include things such as walking and dancing. Although swimming is an excellent exercise for people with osteoarthritis, it is not especially helpful in maintaining bone density because not much weight is placed on the spine or leg bones while swimming.

Specific back exercises are helpful, as long as they are performed without causing strain on the spine. Extension and back stretching exercises are the best to do. These exercises are designed to condition the muscles of the back that pull on the vertebrae. It is this pull of the muscles on the vertebrae, in combination with weight bearing, that leads to increased bone formation. A back extension exercise is included in Chapter 5 (see "Back Extension," page 76).

Types of Exercises and Activities to Avoid

Flexion exercises of the back, in which the back is bent forward, increase the risk of fracture by compressing the front of the vertebrae. Therefore, if you have advanced osteoporosis, flexion exercises such as the partial sit-up described in Chapter 3 should be avoided. When doing any exercise, stretch only to the point where you can feel the stretch, not to the point of causing pain.

People who already have osteoporosis should avoid heavy weight-lifting activities with their arms. Lifting heavy weights greatly increases the stress on vertebrae which are already fragile. Using light one- or two-pound weights as resistance for exercises is fine, but using heavier weights should be avoided.

Calcium

Calcium is a major component of bone and is necessary for normal bone formation. A diet high in calcium can help slow down the process of bone loss. It is recommended that men and premenopausal women get 1000 milligrams of pure calcium per day and that postmenopausal women get 1500 milligrams per day.

Diet and Calcium

Eating a varied diet that is rich in dairy products is the best way to obtain adequate calcium. However, most people do not get enough calcium in their normal diets. The average American woman gets only 50% of the recommended daily allowance of calcium from diet alone. Because it so hard to get all the calcium needed from diet alone, most doctors recommend that postmenopausal women take daily calcium supplements.

Calcium Supplements

Calcium is usually supplemented in the form of calcium carbonate tablets that you can purchase in most pharmacies and health food stores. Calcium carbonate also is available as oyster shell calcium and as a major ingredient in some antacid medications. Some frozen orange juice concentrates also are fortified with calcium. Multivitamins contain a small amount of calcium, but usually not enough to ensure an adequate daily supply.

All preparations of calcium carbonate contain about 40% pure calcium. If your recommended amount of calcium is 1500 mg per day, you will need to take a little over 3000 mg of calcium carbonate to get the required amount of pure calcium. Usually the only side effect you might encounter from calcium supplements is mild constipation. However, if you have a history of kidney stones, you should consult your physician before taking calcium. For some people, calcium can increase the risk of developing more kidney stones.

Vitamin D

Vitamin D is needed in order for your body to use calcium effectively to form new bone. Vitamin D is obtained in two ways, through diet and sunlight. Dietary sources of Vitamin D include fortified milk, fatty fish, chicken liver, and egg yolk. Americans generally have diets adequate in Vitamin D and get enough exposure to the sun so that they do not need Vitamin D supplements. However, some elderly people can have a mild Vitamin D deficiency due to insufficient diet and lack of exposure to sunlight.

As a precaution, it is recommended that all elderly people take one multivitamin daily. There are no side effects to taking a daily multivitamin, and you can be certain you are receiving an adequate supply of most vitamins, including Vitamin D.

Medical Treatments

Your physician may prescribe medications for the treatment of osteoporosis or compression fractures. The most

commonly used medication is estrogen, which is prescribed for women after menopause.

Estrogen

Several studies have found that estrogen helps slow the
loss of bone and decreases the risk of fractures. It cannot,
however, restore bone that has already been lost. Estrogen
works most effectively on the bones of the back. It also has been shown to provide some protection to the
hip bones.

Estrogen is most beneficial when started early after
menopause. This is because bone loss is the most rapid, and
most preventable, during the first years after menopause.
The effect of estrogen appears to be strongest when it is
used in conjunction with calcium. Therefore, if you are taking estrogen, it is especially important to make sure you are
also getting adequate calcium.

Not only is estrogen very helpful in preventing osteoporosis, it also may offer some protection against heart
attacks in some older women. Like any drug, at times,
estrogen may have harmful side effects. Consultation
with your physician can help you weigh the risks and
benefits of using estrogen.

Estrogen is not indicated for everyone with osteoporosis.
Other medical treatments are available, and new thera-
pies are being developed. Your physician can advise you
which medications may be appropriate for you.

Summary

Prevention is the best treatment for osteoporosis. However, if you already have the disease, there are still things you can do to limit its progression and to decrease the risk of developing fractures. Along with eating a balanced diet and taking calcium supplementation if needed, remaining active and mobile is one of the keys to preserving bone density and preventing fractures.

Chapter 10

Common Conditions and Drugs Affecting Mobility

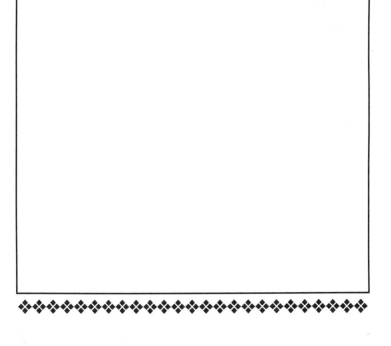

Acute Illness

Sometimes a slight decline in functioning or mobility is the first sign of an infection or new heart condition for an older person.

Infection

Acute illnesses such as pneumonia, bladder infections, and flu all can start out with the same symptoms. It may take you longer to get out of bed and get moving in the morning, or stair climbing may make you feel more short of breath. You may notice a lack of energy and pep. If you have been previously self-sufficient, but suddenly need help with your normal daily routine or basic home-making tasks, you may be suffering from a new infection.

New Heart Condition

Sometimes an abrupt change in functioning indicates a new cardiac condition such as heart failure or a heart attack. Your only symptom of a new heart problem may be shortness of breath with activities that normally would not be a problem for you. You will not necessarily have pain with a heart ailment.

What You Can Do

It is important to consult your physician when you notice a sudden decline in your mobility. Sometimes minor symptoms can signify major medical problems. A telephone call to keep your doctor informed of any changes in your health may prevent an acute illness from becoming life-threatening.

Dehydration

Older people are more likely to have problems with dehydration than younger people. This is due primarily to the fact that when you get older your thirst mechanism is not as sensitive. Therefore, you may not have the sensation of being thirsty, even though your body is becoming dehydrated.

One of the primary symptoms of dehydration is a lack of energy. This can occur gradually over a day or two and may present itself as a slow loss of strength and mobility. Feeling dizzy when first standing up from sitting or lying down is another common symptom of dehydration. People are at a much greater risk for falling when they are dehydrated.

What You Can Do

Drinking lots of fluids is the key to preventing dehydration. Fluids include all kinds of liquids, such as water, juice, milk, soup, and soda. It is best to avoid caffeinated beverages such as coffee and tea, however, because they can worsen dehydration by increasing urination.

If you don't have a problem with fluid retention, such as swelling of your feet or ankles or congestive heart failure, your diet should include 8 glasses of fluids a day. If the weather is hot or if you have been physically active, you need to drink even more fluids. If you have problems with fluid retention, your doctor can advise you on the appropriate amount of fluids to drink. To find out more about fluid retention, see the section on congestive heart failure at the end of this chapter.

Alcohol

People often do not think of alcohol as a drug, but indeed it is a drug that has very strong effects on the brain and nervous system. Even a small amount of alcohol can slow reaction time and impair balance. Tolerance for alcohol decreases with age. This means it takes less alcohol to cause negative effects in an older person compared to a younger person.

Alcohol is a particularly dangerous drug for people who already have problems with mobility. The risk of falling and injuring yourself is greatly increased if you have problems with mobility and consume alcohol. People who have memory problems are also at increased risk for the negative effects of alcohol. Because alcohol affects the brain, thinking and judgment are further impaired when you use alcohol.

What You Can Do

If you choose to drink alcohol, be certain to do so in moderation. The effects of alcohol on coordination and reaction time can last up to a full day! Remember, you need to be extra cautious with walking and moving around whenever you drink, even if it is only one glass of wine or beer.

Blood Pressure Medications

High blood pressure in and of itself should not affect your mobility. However, some of the medications used to treat high blood pressure may have side effects that impair your mobility. Some blood pressure medications lead to fatigue because they slow down the pumping action of the heart. You may notice that it takes you a little longer to climb steps or get up and dressed in the morning after you start taking a new blood pressure medication.

Several of the blood pressure medications can cause your blood pressure to drop too low, particularly when you first stand up from lying down or sitting. If your blood pressure drops too low, you may feel dizzy or faint when you first stand up. Other blood pressure medications called diuretics (water pills) sometimes can lead to dehydration, and this also can result in dizziness.

What You Can Do

If You Feel Fatigued

If your blood pressure medicine is causing you to feel more fatigued, you can compensate by slowing down your gait, particularly on stairs and hills. You still should be able to exercise, however, even if you are on a medication that is decreasing your heart's pumping action. If you feel the medication you are taking is slowing you down too much, talk to your doctor to find out if another blood pressure medicine can be substituted.

If You Feel Dizzy

If you have a problem with getting dizzy when you stand up, there are several things you can do. Start by moving your feet up and down several times before you stand up. This will help pump the blood up from your legs toward your head. When you first get up, stand by the chair or bed for a minute before you start walking. This will allow the lightheadedness to resolve before you move. You also can try marching in place when you first stand up. This activity will help move the blood toward your head.

If dizziness continues to be a problem, see your doctor. Perhaps a different blood pressure medication would be better suited for you. Your doctor also may recommend wearing special support stockings which help pump the blood back toward your heart. Additional information on what you can do if you feel dizzy is provided in Chapter 7.

Other Medications

Many common prescription and nonprescription drugs affect mobility. Any medication that causes drowsiness or affects thinking ability can affect mobility. Sedatives, medications used to treat depression, and pain relievers that contain codeine, morphine, or other narcotics are categories of drugs that often impair function and mobility. Also, many over-the-counter allergy medicines, such as Allerest®, Contac®, Benadryl®, and Actifed® have sleepiness as a side effect and therefore may impair your mobility.

What You Can Do

If you have a problem walking or tend to lose your balance, you should discuss the drugs you are taking with your doctor. You may be experiencing side effects from your medications. Sometimes one drug alone does not cause a problem, but several drugs taken in combination may interact and affect your mobility. Also, be sure to tell your doctor about any over-the-counter drugs you are taking. Even nonprescription medications can alter your gait or sense of balance.

Vision Problems that Affect Mobility

Cataracts

Cataracts commonly occur as people age. Fifteen percent of all people over the age of 50 develop cataracts. The lens of the eye becomes cloudy, and there is a gradual decrease in vision. Problems with glare are one of the first things people notice as cataracts form.

What You Can Do

Slow your walking pace if you are having trouble seeing. You want to be sure of yourself and notice any obstacles that may be in your way. Be particularly careful when you are in unfamiliar surroundings or on uneven ground.

If you are bothered by glare, you should move even more cautiously when there is a high gloss floor surface such as a waxed and polished floor. Excessively bright light and direct sunlight also make glare more noticeable. Soft, shaded lighting is the best for limiting glare.

Medical Treatment

Be sure to consult your physician if you notice a change in your vision or if you begin to have more trouble with glare. Frequently, surgery will be recommended if a cataract is significant enough to cause you trouble walking. Most often an artificial lens is implanted during surgery to replace the clouded one. With surgery and lens implantation your vision can be restored to very close to what it was before the cataract developed.

Glaucoma

Another fairly common disease for older people is glaucoma. In this disease, the pressure inside the eye increases and eventually pinches off the nerves from the eye to the brain. Peripheral vision, what you see on the edges of your field of vision, is lost first. As glaucoma gets worse, you develop tunnel vision so that you are able to see only the very center of your normal visual field. This is like looking through a long tube, or tunnel, where you cannot see anything to either side.

What You Can Do

There are several things you can do to cope with the loss of vision due to glaucoma. When you walk, you can compensate for the loss of peripheral vision by turning your head more often to see things on either side. Keep objects and clutter out of the pathways where you walk around your home. As with cataracts, if you walk somewhat more slowly and generally more cautiously, you will be less likely to fall from tripping or running into things you do not see.

Medical Treatment

If you have loss of vision due to glaucoma, unfortunately there is no cure. However, prescription eye drops are available which can prevent or delay the progression of the disease. An ophthalmologist can determine if such eye drops would be beneficial for you.

Age-Related Macular Degeneration

Age-related macular degeneration is a common eye condition that occurs as people get older. For many people it causes no problems with vision at all. However, for some people, macular degeneration causes significant vision loss. Age-related macular degeneration is a major cause of blindness in people over age 65 in the United States. Vision distortion, or things appearing out of focus, is often an early symptom.

What You Can Do

If you have some loss of vision from macular degeneration, the most important thing you can do is to develop ways of adapting so you can remain mobile. Using good lighting helps by providing the most illumination possible. You also may want to use a cane to give you extra stability walking.

You can consult a low vision specialist to obtain further information about specific aids in coping with impaired vision. *Coping With Low Vision*, another book in the Coping with Aging Series, gives you detailed information about aids to help you adapt if your vision is impaired.

Medical Treatment

Age-related macular degeneration is sometimes treatable if detected early, before there is a significant loss of vision. Therefore it is important to get regular eye exams as you get older so that macular degeneration and other eye conditions can be discovered and treated as early as possible. Although not a therapy for everyone, treatment with laser surgery is helpful in certain cases.

Dementia

Believe it or not, you need to think about walking when you walk. There are numerous hazards in the environment that can affect your safety when you are walking. You need to be, at least on a subconscious level, aware of the cracks in the sidewalk, the height of steps, and other obstacles in your surroundings.

You probably do not realize it, but on some level you should be constantly paying attention to where you place your feet and to what is around you as you take each step. It is harder for people with dementia to pay attention to their surroundings. Because of this they are more likely to stumble or trip.

Alzheimer's disease is the most common type of dementia affecting older adults. Dementia and Alzheimer's disease are discussed in detail in *Coping with Alzheimer's Disease and Other Dementing Illnesses*, another book in the Coping with Aging Series.

As dementia progresses, walking sometimes becomes more and more difficult as the gait pattern changes. Often, movements become slower, steps are shorter, and balance is impaired. Posture can become bent-over, and mobility may be further limited by a decrease in flexibility.

One of the tragedies of dementia is that people quit walking. This can lead to a downward spiral of complications as people develop breathing problems and further weakness as a result of being less active. Pressure ulcers or bed sores can develop once someone is no longer up and moving around.

What You Can Do

It is important for people with dementia to continue to walk as much as possible. Keeping the environment free of clutter and obstacles will help ensure safety while the person remains active. Using a cane or walker can help a person with Alzheimer's disease remain steady when walking. Chapter 13 gives more information on how to choose a cane or walker. In later stages of the disease, the person may need supervision to walk safely. The main thing is to allow the person with dementia to remain active and mobile for as long as possible.

Medical Treatment

Unfortunately, in most cases, dementia cannot be cured. However, sometimes symptoms of forgetfulness or confusion are not due to dementia but to depression or another medical problem. A thorough medical examination is important to determine the cause of the symptoms.

Parkinson's Disease

Parkinson's disease is a condition in which a particular part of the brain, known as the basal ganglia, degenerates. This disease leads to characteristic problems of gait, mobility, and posture. Movements generally become slow, and it becomes especially difficult to start a motion. It may take a long time to get up from a chair or get out of a car. People may have a hard time taking the first few steps when walking. Ironically, once walking has begun, the gait often gets progressively faster and faster, and it then becomes difficult to stop or change directions.

Balance also is affected by Parkinson's disease. Normally, people have a very finely tuned sense of balance so that small adjustments to posture are constantly being made to stay upright. With Parkinson's disease, people have trouble making these adjustments, and it is easy for them to lose their balance and fall.

What You Can Do

Joint stiffness often becomes a problem in Parkinson's disease. The flexibility exercises described in Chapter 5 are a good starting point for a stretching program. Because fatigue also is also a common problem with this illness, exercises should be done frequently, but for short periods of time. Stretching in a chair, then getting up and taking a short walk is a simple exercise format that is not too fatiguing.

Medical Treatment

Many medications are used to treat Parkinson's disease. You should have regular medical follow-up to have your condition monitored and your medications adjusted.

Physical and occupational therapy are extremely important if you have Parkinson's disease. A therapist can design an individualized program with specific exercises related to the mobility problems caused by the illness. Therapists also can recommend modifications of your home environment so you can remain as mobile as possible. Chapter 14 contains more information on home adaptations. Finally, a physical therapist also may instruct you in the use of a cane or a type of walker to allow you to continue walking. Remaining active for as long as possible is a goal that cannot be stressed too much.

Stroke

A stroke is damage to the brain resulting from one of two causes: rupture or blockage of a blood vessel in the brain. With either of these events, some brain cells die and the brain loses some of its capacities. The degree of mobility impairment following a stroke depends on what part of the brain has been affected. Disability resulting from damage to the brain can range from very mild, with no noticeable long-term loss in mobility, to a severe loss of function affecting one or both sides of the body. Other problems resulting from a stroke can include difficulties with speech, vision, judgment, or memory.

If a stroke involves the part of the brain that controls leg strength, you certainly will have difficulty with mobility. Also the side of the body with muscle weakness over time usually becomes stiffer, making your leg and trunk movement less agile and walking more difficult. Sometimes, however, even if your strength is normal your sensation, coordination, or balance may be impaired. If this is the case, your mobility can be affected even if muscle weakness is not a problem.

Another common problem after a stroke is neglect of one side of the body. When this happens, a person becomes less aware of one leg or arm, or not as mindful of where it is in space. If someone is not aware of where their leg or foot is as they take a step, walking can be very difficult. Also, safety is a real concern with neglect because the chances of mis-stepping and falling are greatly increased.

What You Can Do

If you have had a stroke that resulted in muscle weakness, walking requires a lot more energy. Most likely, you will fatigue easily after walking relatively short distances. Therefore, you need to take frequent short rests and plan activities to allow rest times. When planning a walk, choose a place where there will be benches or chairs along the way. Shopping trips may need to be short, and it is best to shop at times when there is not a lot of congestion or long lines.

Exercises

After a stroke, it is important to keep your muscles as limber as possible. This is best done by remaining active and following an exercise program. Make sure some of your exercises involve fully stretching the muscles and moving the joints as far as possible to maintain flexibility. Chapter 5 has a number of stretching exercises you can choose from.

Some of your exercises also should be aimed at strengthening the muscles. Strengthening exercises, such as those described in Chapter 3, can help counteract some of the weakness resulting from a stroke. Finally, you should include exercises designed to increase your endurance. Chapter 6 gives recommendations on exercises for increasing stamina.

A stroke affects each person in a unique way; therefore you really need an exercise program that is customized for you. You should consult your doctor or see a physical therapist before beginning any new exercise. They can help design the best exercise program for you.

Medical Treatment

Medical treatment for a stroke often involves the use of aspirin or another type of blood thinner. These medications are prescribed to prevent future strokes. Another important part of stroke treatment is controlling blood pressure and avoiding tobacco. In select cases your doctor may recommend surgery to remove blockages in the blood vessels in the neck.

If you have severe leg weakness that causes your foot to drag or slap the floor as you walk, a brace may be prescribed to help keep your foot up. A brace also can help keep your ankle and knee in correct alignment. If a brace is necessary, it should be worn according to the instructions of your therapist.

Heart Disease

Many different cardiac conditions are included under the heading of heart disease.

Angina

Angina, or chest pain caused by a lack of oxygen to the heart, can limit mobility. If you develop angina you may notice you cannot climb as many steps or walk as far as you used to before becoming fatigued or developing chest pain.

The amount of activity done before noticing angina varies from person to person. Some people may be able to walk several blocks before they develop chest pain. Others may experience angina after walking across a room. In general, the earlier the onset of chest pain after starting an activity, the more severe the coronary disease.

What You Can Do

The first thing to do if you develop angina is to stop the activity you are doing and sit down to rest. If you know that a particular activity sometimes causes chest pain, you can pace yourself while doing that activity. By taking frequent short rests you may be able to avoid angina. For example, when you are walking uphill, you can slow down or stop for brief periods to put less of a strain on your heart.

Medical Treatment

Of course, none of these measures is a substitute for seeing your doctor and following medical advice. Your doctor most likely will prescribe medications that allow you to increase your activity level without developing chest pain. Often nitroglycerin is prescribed for you to take when you develop chest pain. Sometimes surgery or angioplasty, a nonsurgical technique used to dilate the blood vessels of the heart, is recommended. Not everyone is a candidate for these procedures, however. You should see your physician to determine the best treatment for you.

Congestive Heart Failure

Congestive heart failure is a condition in which the heart muscle weakens and does not pump blood as effectively as it should. It is a fairly common problem among older people. If you have this condition, you may find that you get short of breath with activity and fatigue easily.

Also with congestive heart failure your blood pressure can sometimes drop too low. If your heart isn't pumping as strongly as it should, your blood may not be moving forcefully enough to keep your blood pressure as high as it should be. A problem with this is that when you stand up from lying down or sitting, your blood pressure may drop even lower, and your brain may temporarily not get enough blood supply. As a result you may feel dizzy.

In addition, with congestive heart failure, you may build up fluid in your feet and legs, and sometimes in your lungs. Swelling in your legs, or edema, can be an early sign that your body is retaining extra water. Fluid retention places added stress on your heart. It also can make you fatigued and make it difficult for you to get around.

What You Can Do

If your feet or legs swell, you should cut back on your activities and rest more. Being less active will allow your heart to pump more effectively. Other helpful tips for managing swelling are found in Chapter 11.

If you have a problem with your blood pressure dropping too low, you need to be extra cautious when you first stand up to prevent falling. After standing for a minute or two, your blood pressure should readjust to what it normally is.

Pacing Yourself. Pacing yourself is the key to remaining mobile if you have congestive heart failure. Plan short, leisurely walks and arrange frequent rest stops during your walks. Walking in a shopping mall can be ideal because there are usually places to sit and rest whenever you need to.

You should do only a little physical activity at a time, especially if it is strenuous. Space your house- or yard work over the day and over the week, rather than trying to do it all at once. There are several energy saving devices that can make housework and other activities less strenuous. An electric broom, for example, can make sweeping a lot more energy efficient and less taxing.

To conserve energy when you are shopping, use a cart for your groceries instead of carrying them in your arms. Even if you have a small number of items, it is a lot less work to push a cart than it is to carry things. You also can use a serving cart for laundry or other objects you need to move around the house.

Medical Treatment

One of the common treatments your doctor may recommend is limiting salt intake. The sodium in salt causes you to retain water. By restricting the amount of salt in your diet, you can help prevent swelling in your feet and ankles. Diuretics, or water pills, often are prescribed to help eliminate excess fluid. Medications also may be prescribed to help your heart pump more forcefully. Close medical follow-up is needed to monitor your disease and possibly adjust your medications.

Claudication

Claudication is a condition where the blood supply to the muscles is compromised. Most often, this does not cause any problems when you are resting, but when you walk your leg muscles need more circulation. If your muscles do not get enough blood supply when you walk, you may develop pain, most often in the calf muscles. The pain is relieved when you stop walking.

What You Can Do

It is important not to stop exercising if you have claudication. In fact, a regular walking program may actually *improve* the circulation in your legs. With training, you may find you can walk a further distance before pain develops. Chapter 6 has information on starting a walking exercise program.

Medical Treatment

If the distance you can walk is limited by calf pain, you should consult your physician. Aspirin or other types of blood thinners may be prescribed to increase the blood supply to your legs. Sometimes medications you are taking for other problems can make claudication worse. Your doctor will review your medications and also make sure your pain is not caused by other conditions.

Lung Diseases

Emphysema, asthma, and bronchitis are the most common lung diseases in the elderly. All of these will affect your mobility to some extent. When you walk you need to get more oxygen to your heart and muscles compared to when you are sitting. With lung disease you often cannot get as much oxygen as you need when you exert yourself. As a result, when you are active you get short of breath and tire easily.

What You Can Do

Just as with heart disease, you need to pace yourself to remain as mobile as possible. When you feel short of breath, stop and rest until your breathing returns to normal. Carrying things adds to the amount of work you do while walking. Using a cart instead of a basket while shopping, and a serving cart to transport items in the kitchen, will decrease the amount of work you do. If you use a walker, having wheels on it will eliminate the work of picking it up. If you are limited in how far you can walk outdoors, an electric scooter may be helpful.

Medical Treatment

If you have lung disease, your doctor may prescribe medications to improve your breathing. Medications that decrease phlegm or open up air passages can allow you to walk further and faster than you did before. In later stages of lung diseases, oxygen may be used to help make breathing easier.

Oxygen Therapy

If you are very short of breath, and provided you don't smoke, oxygen may be prescribed. Because pure oxygen is very flammable it is not prescribed for people who smoke. Oxygen comes in several different forms, some of which are more portable than others. You can explore which form would be best for you with an oxygen vendor.

Home oxygen can be quite expensive and unfortunately is not always covered by Medicare. Your doctor can determine whether you qualify for Medicare reimbursement. Even if you don't receive Medicare or insurance coverage, you may find the investment in home oxygen is well worth the expense in terms of increased energy and mobility.

Diabetes

If you have diabetes, your mobility may be affected in several ways. However, just because you have diabetes does not mean that you necessarily will have impaired mobility. It does mean that you will have to take some basic precautions and be under a physician's care to remain active.

You may have subtle problems with your balance if you have diabetes. The disease often damages the nerves in your legs. This means that your legs and feet may lose some of their feeling. As a result it is harder to feel the ground you are walking on. You also may have trouble knowing where your feet are placed.

Foot problems are a common and potentially very serious problem for people with diabetes. Circulation is compromised as a result of this disease. This means your feet do not get a normal blood supply, and it is harder for a blister or scrape to heal. Also, with compromised circulation, any break in the skin easily can become infected.

What You Can Do

Because you are more prone to foot infections when you have diabetes, it is imperative to wear shoes at all times. It is also important to keep floors clear of objects so you are less likely to bump your feet when you walk.

Be sure to inspect your feet daily so that any minor irritations will be noticed and treated early, before they become infected. Look for areas of swelling or redness or areas where the skin is cracking. Don't forget to check between your toes. Chapter 11 has information on how to deal with foot sores. If a sore doesn't heal within a couple of days, let your doctor know.

Even though you need to take extra caution not to lose your balance or injure your feet if you have diabetes, it is important to remain active. In addition to keeping your heart and muscles conditioned, being active helps keep your blood sugar in good control.

Medical Treatment

One of the major roles your physician plays in managing diabetes is helping control blood sugar either by prescribing oral medications or injections of insulin. A dietician can help you manage your diet, and a therapist can develop an exercise program that will help regulate your blood sugar. Following the advice of your health care providers is particularly important when you have diabetes to prevent as much as possible the complications associated with this disease.

Summary

Whether you have a chronic medical condition or an acute illness, remaining active and mobile is essential to staying as healthy as possible. There are many things you can do to cope with problems of impaired mobility that result from illnesses, from common conditions related to aging, or from medications.

Paying attention to your fluid intake, being extra cautious when you change positions, keeping the floors and stairways clear of obstacles, using a walking aid if recommended, pacing your activities to avoid overfatigue, and consulting with your physician are some of the things you can do to maintain your mobility. Just because you have a chronic medical condition or illness does not mean you have to give up an active lifestyle!

Chapter 11

Feet

Foot pain is a very common cause of mobility problems. Three quarters of active older adults complain of foot pain. Unfortunately, many people are tempted to ignore pain in their feet, even if it affects their walking. This is because they think nothing can be done. Actually, most of the time foot pain is reversible. The cure may be simple, quick, and inexpensive. The disability related to not walking can be just the opposite: complex, long-lasting, and costly.

Cautions Concerning Home Foot Remedies

Check the Sensation in Your Feet

Before doing any home treatment for foot conditions, you should first check to make sure your feet have normal sensation. Take a Q-tip or a cotton ball and pull out a fine wisp of cotton. Gently touch the bottom of the arch of your foot with it. If you can feel the touch of the cotton on your foot, your sensation is probably good enough for you to do home foot treatments such as rubbing calluses with a pumice stone. If you cannot feel the wisp of cotton on your foot, you should not rub down calluses or do other home remedies yourself because you run the risk of inadvertently damaging your skin. In that case you should consult a doctor, nurse, or podiatrist. If you have poor sensation in your feet, you also should get help for routine nail care.

If You Have Poor Vision

If you have poor vision you should not treat calluses or corns yourself. You also should have a health professional do your routine nail care, because you may have trouble trimming your nails adequately.

If You Have Diabetes, Poor Circulation, or Fragile Skin

If you have diabetes, circulation problems, or fragile skin, you should see your doctor or podiatrist as soon as you first notice a callus or corn. Because even harmless looking corns, calluses, and warts can develop into open sores, do *not* attempt to treat them yourself. These should all be treated by a medical professional as soon as they develop. Also, avoid over-the-counter foot medications. They often contain acids which can be too harsh for your fragile skin. The sooner any skin condition of your feet is treated, the better it is for your health and mobility.

If you do notice the start of a sore, it is even more important for you to see your physician promptly. The blood supply to your feet may not be sufficient to allow an open sore to heal. A minor sore may turn into a large ulcer and easily become infected.

It is advisable to have routine nail care done by a nurse or podiatrist if you have diabetes or circulation problems. Professional nail care is the best way to guarantee that cuts or sores do not develop around the ends of your toes where they are most vulnerable to infection.

Skin

Dry Skin

Dry skin is a very common problem for older people. As people age the oil glands in the feet do not work as well as they used to, and the skin becomes drier. This can cause two problems. First, it can cause your feet to become itchy. If you scratch your dry feet, they may become inflamed and susceptible to infection. Second, dry skin can predispose your feet to cracking. This too can cause an infection. If your feet develop an infection, more than likely they will become very painful and sometimes swollen as well. The pain and swelling will make walking difficult.

Self-treatment

Use of a skin cream can help the skin retain moisture. Creams are most effective if applied right after you have bathed, while your skin is still damp. They help lock in the water and keep your skin from drying out.

"Urea-based" lotions are effective in keeping feet from becoming dry and itchy. Check the label on moisturizing lotion to see whether urea is listed as an ingredient. You may need to apply lotion both in the morning and at night to keep your feet from drying out. Soaking your feet in warm (but never hot!) water prior to applying lotion will not do any harm as long as you are sure to apply lotion afterwards.

CAUTION: Simply soaking your feet, without applying moisturizing lotion afterwards, will increase the skin's dryness. This is because water strips the oils off the skin.

Medical Treatment

If itching or dryness do not improve with the frequent use of a moisturizing lotion, you may have a fungal infection, eczema or allergic dermatitis, or another skin condition that requires medical attention. Consult your physician. Treatment frequently involves the use of topical prescription medications.

Callus

A callus is an overgrowth of skin layers which occurs in response to increased friction or pressure on one part of the foot. The most common location of callus formation is on the ball of the foot. Another common location is directly over bunions. Calluses can become worse if your shoes do not fit correctly. This is because poor-fitting shoes can increase friction on one part of your foot.

Self-treatment

Shoes. Treatment of calluses starts with eliminating the cause of the increased friction or pressure. This may mean getting different shoes or slowly breaking in new shoes. Wearing shoes that fit well is critical to preventing calluses. Shoes need to have sufficient padding on the inside and the soles need to be cushioned adequately. Chapter 12 gives more detail about what to look for when buying new shoes.

Pumice Stone and Moisturizing Lotion. For small calluses, you can smooth down the skin build-up yourself using a pumice stone. Rubbing the callus with a pumice stone will gradually wear down the extra skin. When rubbing a callus, you should not be overvigorous, because this may cause you to tear off healthy skin. It is best to take off just a little of the callus at a time. You usually need to work on a callus several times to remove the built-up skin. You may find using a pumice stone is easier after you have first soaked your feet to soften the skin. After using a pumice stone, it is a good idea to always use a cream or lotion to moisturize the skin.

CAUTION: Before using a pumice stone on your feet, please read the information at the beginning of this chapter to make sure you have no contraindication to home treatment of your callus.

Medical Treatment

A podiatrist or other health care provider trained in foot care can shave down calluses for you. Sometimes you also need to see a podiatrist to get specially molded inserts to wear inside your shoes. These inserts add cushioning to the soles of your feet and relieve pressure areas you may have on the bottoms of your feet that are causing calluses.

Corns

Corns are similar to calluses in that they are a build-up of skin. The difference is that a corn is much more concentrated, with a small dense area of skin growth. This

Feet

becomes the core, or center of the corn. They usually occur over a bony deformity of the foot such as a hammer toe (see page 184).

Corns can be either hard or soft. Hard corns tend to occur on the top of the toes where they rub against the shoes. Soft corns tend to occur between the toes where there is pressure of one toe rubbing against another. The reason these corns are soft is because there is more moisture between the toes which keeps the skin soft.

Major problems with corns are twofold. The first problem is they often hurt and make it hard for you to walk. The other problem is that corns can become infected and be difficult to heal. Both of these problems can be addressed either by caring for your corns yourself or seeking medical treatment if home remedies are not advised or are ineffective.

Self-treatment

Shoes. When corns develop it is usually a sign that your shoes do not fit as well as they should. If you have a corn on the top of your toe, it may mean you should be wearing a shoe with more depth. Sometimes "extra-depth shoes" are the best solution. Corns between the toes can mean that your shoes are too narrow. Shoes that are extra-wide across the toes may be helpful in treating this type of corn.

Pumice Stones and Moisturizing Lotion. Treatment of corns is similar to that for calluses. You need to smooth down the overgrown skin with a pumice stone. However, with corns this is more difficult to do than it is with calluses. Using a skin moisturizer on corns usually is of some help. Moisturizers aid in preventing the skin around a corn from breaking open and becoming infected.

CAUTION: Before attempting to treat your corn with a pumice stone, you should read the section at the beginning of the chapter to be sure you have no contraindication to self-treatment.

Protective Padding. The other part of treatment for corns is applying protective padding around the corn to relieve pressure on the area. For soft corns between your toes, you can use lamb's wool to separate the toes. Lamb's wool generally works better than cotton batting for padding because it compresses less and doesn't wear out as easily. Lamb's wool is inexpensive and odor free. It can be purchased from well-stocked pharmacies or medical supply stores. For hard corns protective pads can be purchased at most pharmacies. They come in two types. One has a central precut hole designed to fit over the corn. The other type is shaped like a horseshoe, with the corn sitting in the center of the opening. In general use whichever type is more comfortable for you. However, if you have poor circulation the horseshoe corn pad is safer because it is less likely to restrict circulation.

CAUTION: It is best to avoid pads with medication, because these may injure the normal skin around the corn. Also, if you have diabetes, fragile skin, or circulation problems, pads with adhesive backs should not be used. Removing adhesive-backed pads can sometimes break open the skin and you may have trouble healing an open sore.

Medical Treatment

If a corn recurs frequently or persists for a long time and interferes with your walking, you should consult your physician or podiatrist. This is for two reasons. The first is that a physician or podiatrist can use a special knife to remove your corn. The second is that they can prescribe specially molded shoes or shoe inserts to relieve pressure over corns.

Unfortunately, if a corn is soft and is associated with an underlying bony deformity, it may be very difficult to cure without surgery. As long as the bony pressure point exists, the corn will recur. Your physician may recommend surgery to correct the underlying foot deformity that is leading to the corn formation. However, surgery may not be the best course for all older people. There are always some risks, such as infection or a nonhealing sore, resulting from surgery. In addition, surgery will keep you off your feet for a while, so your mobility will decline temporarily.

Warts

Warts may look similar to corns but they are caused by viruses, and are not the result of pressure areas. Warts on the feet usually are not permanent. After an average of 4 or 5 months they tend to disappear on their own. If the warts are painless they do not need to be treated at all. It is only when warts spread or cause pain that interferes with walking that they need to be treated.

Self-treatment

Treatment involves smoothing down of the wart with a pumice stone and applying an over-the counter wart removal medication. Medication should be applied following the specific instructions on the container. You should to be careful when you apply it so that you do not get the medication on normal skin.

CAUTION: Before treating *any* wart yourself you should check with your physician to make sure that what you have is a wart. You also need to ensure you do not have any underlying health problems that could make home treatment dangerous.

Medical Treatment

In some cases, painful warts will not go away with simple treatment and may need to be "burned off." This is done in a physician's office by applying a strong chemical to the wart which kills the skin that contains the virus causing the wart.

Foot Sores

It is extremely important for you to be aware of the skin condition of your feet. When you are older, the tissues of your feet do not get as much blood supply, the skin becomes thinner, and if a sore develops it is harder to heal. You need to be very careful not to injure your feet or to let corns or calluses get out of hand. A minor scrape or bump on your toe will take longer to heal when you are older compared to when you were young.

Treatment

Because it is so important for keeping active, taking care of your feet is critical so that you will not need to stop walking to help heal an ulcer. It is recommended that you inspect your feet daily. If you notice a sore spot, see your podiatrist or physician.

Nails

Approximately one third of older people report painful toenails. Unfortunately, nail pain can make walking very difficult. Pain in the toenails usually is due to one of three things: overly long nails, overgrowth of the nail bed on the side of the nail, or an ingrown toenail. Almost always, these problems can be prevented by good routine nail care.

Routine Nail Care

Nails are best maintained if they are kept at a length that extends just slightly beyond the skin. Toenails should be trimmed with a large toenail clipper to ensure that the nail is cut evenly all the way across. Nails grow at different rates so there are no firm guidelines as to how often they require trimming.

CAUTION: Many older people have trouble doing routine nail care. It can be very difficult, or impossible, to trim your toenails if you are not limber enough to sit and position your foot so you can reach your nails. Also, as

you get older nails thicken and become much more difficult to cut. Older people who have trouble trimming
their nails should get routine foot care from another person such as a nurse, trained bath aid, or podiatrist.

Overgrowth of the Nail Bed

Many people have pain at the side edges of the nail and
this often is mistaken for an ingrown toenail. Pain at the
side of the nail is most likely due to an overgrowth of the
nail bed. This results in a callus formation where the nail
meets the skin. Pressure from the toenail on this skin callus causes the pain. In response to the pressure, the nail
itself becomes thicker, harder, and curves inward.

Treatment

Treatment of an overgrown nail bed involves grinding
down the thickened nail. This usually requires special
tools and is best done by a podiatrist. Sometimes the
margin of the nail needs to be removed as well. Despite
the trouble and cost of seeing a podiatrist, correcting nail
pain is well worth it if it allows you to keep walking.

Ingrown Nails

A nail that is cut too short on the sides, or is uneven, can
press down as it grows and actually grow into the skin.
This results in a painful ingrown toenail. Infection sometimes occurs around the ingrown nail, and this can further increase the pain and pressure in your toe.

Treatment

Treatment for an infected ingrown nail almost always requires minor surgery to remove the embedded part of the nail. This surgery usually can be done in a physician's or podiatrist's office. The best way to prevent ingrown nails is to trim the nails with a toenail clipper so that they are cut evenly and straight across.

Fungal Infections

Fungal infections of toenails cause them to grow thicker and often unevenly. The nails appear discolored and scarred. These infections occur fairly frequently in older people. Fungal infections in and of themselves are not painful, but they may cause impaired mobility. When an enlarged and thickened nail rubs against the shoe, discomfort and problems walking can result.

Treatment

There are three important treatments you can do if you have a fungal infection of your toenails. The most important treatment is to keep the nails clipped and ground down so that the nail bed is not irritated by your shoes pressing against the thick nail. Nails can be ground thinner using a sturdy, rigid, large emery board.

CAUTION: Before clipping or grinding down your nails yourself be sure to read the section on contraindications to self-treatment at the beginning of this chapter.

The second most important thing to do is to make sure your shoes have plenty of room in the toes, so the nails don't rub against the shoes when you walk. You may need to purchase extra-depth or extra-width shoes if ordinary shoes are not large enough.

The third treatment you can do is to apply an antifungal ointment at the margins of the nail to help keep the tissue soft. Some of these preparations are available without a prescription; others are prescribed by your doctor.

Bones

Bunions and Bunionettes

One quarter of older people with painful feet have bunions. A bunion is an overgrowth of the bone at the base of the big toe. A bunionette is an overgrowth of bone at the base of the little toe (see the illustration on the next page).

Bunions and bunionettes can cause pain and difficulty walking if the area over the bony overgrowth becomes inflamed. This can happen if there is pressure from the shoe rubbing over the bone. Bunions also can cause pain if the big toe shifts as a result of the bunion and drifts under the second toe. This causes the second toe to be pushed up, resulting in a painful hammer toe.

Self-treatment

The most important treatment that you can do for bunions and bunionettes is to keep pressure off the bony over-

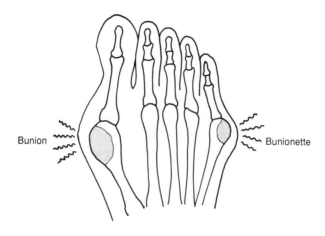

Bunion · Bunionette

Bunion and bunionette.

growth. This is done by wearing shoes that are wide enough to accommodate the bunion or bunionette. Shoes you already own can be cut out over the appropriate area to relieve the pressure of a bunion or bunionette. When you buy new shoes, you should select shoes that are extra wide across the toe and forefoot to keep pressure off these areas. Some people need to purchase custom-molded shoes so they are wide enough to accommodate the bunion or bunionette. To get these shoes, which are specially formed to fit your feet, you need a prescription from a physician or podiatrist.

Medications such as Tylenol®, aspirin, and other anti-inflammatory drugs may help treat the pain of a bunion or bunionette. Chapter 8 provides more information on pain-relieving medications. If you need to take any of these medications more than once or twice a week, you should notify your doctor.

Medical Treatment

It is important to remember that medical treatments for bunions and bunionettes are not substitutes for wearing footwear that is wide enough to relieve pressure over the area. However, medical treatments do play a role in relieving the pain associated with these conditions.

Your doctor may treat painful bunions or bunionettes with prescription medication or with injections. Various anti-inflammatory drugs which are similar to aspirin and ibuprofen are available by prescription. Sometimes these are effective when Tylenol® and aspirin are not.

Acute inflammation of a bunion or bunionette sometimes is treated by a physician injecting the area over the bunion with a medication to reduce swelling and relieve pain. The only true cure for either a bunion or bunionette is surgery, but this is indicated only when there is significant impairment of mobility or excessive pain. Surgery is not necessary purely for cosmetic reasons.

Hammer Toes

Hammer toes are bony, claw-like deformities of the toes. They usually occur on the second through fifth toes. The affected toe becomes permanently bent at the joint. This causes two problems. First, the toe joint is bent up so that it rides higher in the shoe than normal. This results in excessive pressure from the top of the shoe on the hammer toe joint. This can be quite painful. Second, the tip of the toe becomes bent downward so that it presses into the bottom of the shoe. This too often causes pain. Eventually corns can develop over both of these pressure points, the top of the hammer toe and the tip of the toe (see the illustration below).

Self-treatments

Toe Pad. Treatment of a hammer toe is aimed at reducing pressure on the joint and on the tip of the toe. Different types of pads may be used for this purpose. Some are made of foam; others are made of moleskin which is a thin, felt-like material. Foam pads are available either with or without adhesive backing while moleskin always has an adhesive backing. Foam or moleskin pads may be purchased at well-stocked pharmacies or

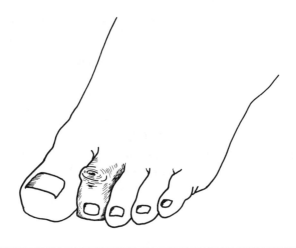

Hammer toe.

shoe stores. One type of pad is not necessarily better than another, and choice of a particular pad depends on what works best for you.

Foam or moleskin pads are placed on the toe to take pressure off the pressure points. Pads should be cut to the desired size and shape to fit the toe. You may need to cut out a hole in the pad to place over the affected area of the hammer toe. What you are doing is building up material around the raised toe joint to relieve the pressure on the painful area itself.

CAUTION: If you have diabetes, fragile skin, or circulation problems, it is best not to use pads with adhesive backs. Removing adhesive backed pads can sometimes break open the skin and you may have trouble healing an open sore.

Lamb's Wool. Lamb's wool also is frequently used to relieve the pressure areas from hammer toes. It can be wrapped around a single toe or woven between toes to relieve the pressure of one toe on another.

The Correct Shoes. An important aspect of treatment is proper footwear. The key is to find shoes that do not put pressure on your hammer toes. Sometimes it is difficult to find shoes with sufficient depth so that they do not rub on the hammer toes. If this is the case, you may need to purchase extra-depth shoes. These are shoes that have increased height in the toe area to accommodate the hammer toe. Shoe stores that cater to customers with hard to fit feet usually carry extra-depth shoes.

Medical Treatments

If lamb's wool, padding, and extra-depth shoes are not effective in relieving pain and allowing you to walk as much as you would like, you should consult a podiatrist or physician. Surgery may be recommended. Sometimes cutting the tendon that is causing the hammer toe is all that is needed. This simple procedure can be done in a physician's or podiatrist's office under a local anesthetic. Sometimes, however, the bones around the joint also need to be reshaped. This involves a more extensive surgical procedure, but it too can usually be done without staying overnight in a hospital. If at all possible, simple surgeries that allow you to get up and move around sooner, rather than later, are preferred.

Joints

Osteoarthritis of the Toe

Arthritis involving the big toe joint is as common as arthritis of the hip or knee joint. As the disease progresses the bones of the toe overgrow and can lead to a frozen joint. The big toe becomes rigid and does not bend. This makes walking awkward, interferes with balance reactions, and frequently is painful.

Self-treatment

Soaks. Soaking your feet in warm water without Epsom salt or other additives may provide pain relief. Be certain that the water is not too hot and be sure to apply a moisturizing lotion generously afterwards. The lotion will help keep your skin from drying out.

CAUTION: Hot Epsom salt soaks is one home remedy for relieving toe joint pain that you should avoid. Part of the problem with using hot soaks is that as you age, your feet do not detect heat as well as when you were young. Because of this, you run the risk of damaging your skin from too much heat. The other problem is that the salts are drying to the skin. When you get older your feet tend to be dry already. Epsom salt soaks can cause excessively dry skin.

Exercises. Joint range of motion exercises can be helpful if the joint is not completely frozen. Bend your toes up and down, and curl your toes under by clawing them. Do this several times a day. Another exercise is to sit in a comfortable chair so your bare feet easily touch the floor and practice picking up a piece of tissue paper with your toes. This exercise forces you to bend and straighten your toe joints.

Shoe Modification. If walking is limited because of toe joint pain or stiffness, having the sole of your shoe stiffened so it does not bend at the big toe may be helpful. A shoe repair shop can add a thin rigid sole to the bottom of your shoes. The sole of your shoe can also be modified with a "rocker bottom." This rigid sole is shaped so that it allows you to roll over the front of your foot as you walk (see the illustration on the next page).

You should see a podiatrist or physician before having your shoes modified with a rocker bottom. Your doctor will write a prescription for the shoe modification. Take this prescription to an orthotist or pedorthist, professionals who design and fit therapeutic footwear. Look in the telephone book yellow pages under "orthopedic appli-

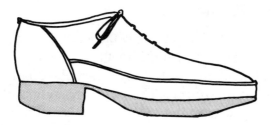

Rocker bottom shoe.

ances" or "shoes—custom made" to find a specialist who can modify your shoes.

Pain Medications. Medications such as Tylenol®, aspirin, and ibuprofen, which commonly are used for pain relief in arthritis involving other joints, may help the big toe joint as well. You may buy many of these over the counter. However, if you find you need to use them more than once or twice a week for toe pain, you should consult your physician.

Medical Treatment

Your physician may prescribe one of a number of medications related to aspirin and ibuprofen. These may be effective even if aspirin or ibuprofen is not. See the section on medications for arthritis, in Chapter 8, for more information about these medications. In addition to prescribing medication, sometimes a physician will inject an arthritic toe joint with a steroid medication, which is a strong anti-inflammatory drug used to relieve pain.

Gout and Pseudogout

All of your joints, but especially the joint of your big toe, can develop a type of arthritis that comes and goes. Gout and pseudogout are the two most common types of this unique form of arthritis. The classic symptoms of gout and pseudogout are a hot and red toe joint. Both diseases are characterized by crystals that form around and in the joint. The difference between gout and pseudogout is in the type of crystal found in the joint.

If you have ever had gout or pseudogout, you know that it is quite painful and can affect your mobility. A big problem is that both conditions tend to recur. One episode may last several weeks and then go away. You may not have another attack for several years or you may have repeated attacks every several months.

Self-treatment

If you have the classic symptoms of gout or pseudogout, home remedies most likely will not be effective. Home remedies include things such as lotions, ointments, and soaks. Because home treatment is ineffective, and because gout symptoms are so painful, you will almost certainly need to see your doctor.

Medical Treatment

Your doctor may draw a sample of fluid from the involved joint and examine it under the microscope to make sure you do not have an infection. Inflammation from gout or pseudogout can be treated by medications injected into the joint or taken by mouth. Sometimes the joint will be injected with steroid medications to relieve pain and inflammation. Treatment is most successful if started early in an attack. Seeing a doctor early during a gout or pseudogout attack will allow you to continue walking as much as possible.

Heel Pain

Heel pain can be caused by a variety of different factors. One of these factors is loss of the fat pad. Thinning of the fat pad is a normal part of growing older. With less cushioning over the heel bone, you are more likely to have heel pain with walking and standing. Frequently heel pain associated with loss of the fat pad gets better after the first few steps, but generally it is worse in the evening after you have been on your feet all day. Heel pain may interfere with your ability to complete even simple daily chores.

Heel pain also may be caused by the presence of a heel spur. This is an overgrowth of the bottom of the heel bone where the arch of the foot begins. Sometimes both a heel spur and loss of the fat pad are present together.

Another cause of heel pain is plantar fascitis. With plantar fascitis, the arch of the foot becomes tense and inflamed at the point where the arch is anchored to the heel at the bottom of the foot. It is often associated with a heel spur. Plantar fascitis may cause pain in the heel or under the arch of the foot. Regardless of the location of pain, plantar fascitis is treated the same way.

Self-treatment

Treatment for loss of the fat pad, heel spurs, and plantar fascitis usually starts with use of a shoe heel cup. A heel cup is a molded plastic insert that is placed inside the heel of your shoe to relieve pressure over the bone of your heel. Plastic heel cups can be purchased from many shoe stores. If use of a heel cup is effective, pain relief should be noticed after using it for several weeks.

Medical Treatment

If pain remains after using a heel cup for several weeks, you should see your physician or podiatrist. For plantar fascitis, if use of heel cup alone is not effective, various types of arch supports may be tried. However, you should consult your physician or podiatrist before you add arch supports to your shoes. Excessive strain in your foot can result if you get an improperly fitting arch support. This can alter the way you walk and lead to pain in other joints and muscles. Injections of steroids and anesthetic medications into the heel also may be used to treat heel pain.

Your physician or podiatrist also can evaluate the way you walk to see if you have a structural problem such as flat feet. Problems with your foot structure may affect your walking and cause you to have persistent or recurrent heel pain. Many times these structural problems can be easily fixed with special shoe modifications.

Forefoot Pain

As with heel pain, there can be a variety of causes of forefoot pain. Forefoot pain is a generalized ache or soreness directly under the ball of the foot.

Morton's Neuroma

Morton's neuroma is an irritation of the nerves in the forefoot. The nerve that travels under the bones of the ball of the foot and connects to the third and fourth toes is usually affected. Sometimes the nerve becomes trapped between these bones and causes pain in the ball of the foot. At times this pain radiates into the toes or even up into the leg. The pain is aggravated by walking. In fact, for some people the pain is so severe that walking becomes almost impossible. Taking your shoes off and massaging your foot often helps relieve the pain of Morton's neuroma. Pain also can occur sharply at rest or at night, even when you are not walking or standing.

This nerve irritation can be caused by shoes that do not fit properly, especially shoes that are too narrow in the toes. However, many times the specific cause of Morton's neuroma is not known.

Treatment

Treatment consists of using an insole in your shoes designed to keep the bones in the ball of your foot from moving as you walk. These inserts need to be custom-made and can be prescribed by a podiatrist. Additionally, your physician may inject the irritated nerve with steroids or an anesthetic agent to provide pain relief. Sometimes the injection needs to be repeated periodically if the pain recurs. Surgery to relieve the pressure on the nerve is needed if shoe inserts or injections do not provide enough relief to enable you to be as active as you would like.

Loss of the Fat Pad

Just like with the heel, there is a loss of the fat pad under the ball of the foot as you age. When you walk and shift your weight to the ball of your foot, instead of having the fat pad cushion your weight, the bones must absorb more of the force.

Treatment

Specific inserts in the soles of your shoes may help relieve forefoot pain by providing shock absorption. These inserts may be prescribed by a physician or podiatrist. Your doctor also may inject the painful area with steroid or anesthetic medication.

Cold Feet

One quarter of older people report having cold feet. Usually cold feet are the result of poor circulation. The blood flow to the feet in young people is strong enough to keep the feet warm. Often, as people get older, the blood supply to the feet becomes restricted, and as a result the feet get cold. In addition to being cold, if you have poor circulation, your feet may be pale in color when they are elevated and become red to purple when they are down.

Treatment

An easy treatment for cold feet is moving them! As you exercise your feet with walking, or even just by moving your ankles and toes, you increase the circulation and warm them up. Of course, putting on socks and shoes also helps keep your feet warm. Soaking your cold feet in a bath of warm water also is effective. Putting lotion on your feet after soaking them will help keep the skin soft.

CAUTION: Although wearing heavy socks can be helpful, you need to be sure they are not too tight or so thick that your shoes do not fit properly. Also, when soaking your feet, you need to be sure the water is not too hot by testing the temperature with your finger before you submerge your feet. Do not use salts or soaps in the water because these may cause your skin to become excessively dry.

Swelling

Swelling of the feet is a very common problem for older people. It can be caused by many things. One of the most common causes is poor blood return from the legs. The veins in the lower legs carry the blood from the feet back to the heart. When you walk or move your feet, ankles, and lower legs the muscles act to help push the blood up. If you become less active when you get older, the blood is not pumped out of the legs as efficiently when you were younger.

With aging, the valves in your veins do not work as effectively to prevent the blood from settling in your feet and ankles. The body's response to this settling blood is to retain water in your feet. This is called edema. Edema also can be caused by other medical conditions such as heart failure and kidney or liver disease, so it is important to see your doctor to find out why you have edema.

Edema, or water retention, affects your mobility by making walking uncomfortable and by limiting the flexibility of your ankles and feet. Another problem with edema is that the extra water in the tissues makes it harder to heal sores and cuts.

Self-treatment

Elevating and Exercising Your Legs

There are several things you can do to control and reduce swelling in your feet. First of all, keep your legs elevated as much as possible. Rest your feet on a footstool when you are sitting. This helps the blood flow back toward your heart. Another important thing is to use your toe, feet, and leg muscles to help pump the blood out of your feet. While you are sitting with your feet elevated, you can move your ankles up and down and bend and straighten your toes. You also can move your ankles in a circle, first in one direction and then in the other. Repeat each of these movements 10 times, and do this several times per day (see the illustration on page 80).

Limiting Salt

Watching how much salt you use also is important if you have problems with edema. Salt in your diet can cause you to retain water and often contributes to swelling in your feet. Try to limit the amount of table salt you add to your food and be aware of the salt content in packaged and prepared foods so you can avoid foods with a high salt content.

Support Stockings

Wearing support stockings can be very helpful in controlling mild swelling. For women, most brands of nylon hosiery carry a line of stockings that give extra support. Pharmacies also carry special elastic support stockings which are suitable for both men and women. If these don't offer enough support, your physician can prescribe a stronger pressure stocking to control edema.

Medical Treatment

If your edema is not controlled by elevating and exercising your feet, limiting your salt intake, and wearing support stockings, your physician may prescribe a medication for you to take. These "diuretics," or water pills, can be very effective in reducing swelling. However, watching your salt intake is still essential to allow medications to be effective.

Summary

Taking proper care of your feet is critical to maintaining your mobility. If your feet are painful, remaining mobile and active becomes very difficult. The treatments described in this chapter should help you in caring for your feet. Self-treatments are suggested when possible. Often, however, seeking treatment from a physician or podiatrist is recommended. This is because good foot care is so important for your mobility, and serious problems can develop from what seem initially to be minor aches or pains. As discussed in this chapter, most foot pain is treatable, and your mobility often need not be impaired because of foot problems.

Chapter 12

Footwear

The type of shoes you wear can make all the difference between having pain-free mobility and having sore feet. When your feet hurt, you are not going to be able to walk as much as you would otherwise. If your shoes do not fit correctly, any foot problems you have will get worse. On the other hand, shoes that fit correctly can actually help heal foot problems such as calluses and corns. Shoes that fit well will relieve pressure areas that contribute to these problems. A properly fitted pair of shoes may be one of the most important investments you can make toward remaining active.

When to Buy New Shoes

There are three thing you need to pay attention to when deciding if it is time to buy new shoes.

1. How your feet feel

2. The way your feet look

3. The condition of your old shoes

How Your Feet Feel

First, let your feet be the main guide to tell you when it is time to buy new shoes. Pay attention to the way your feet feel inside your shoes. If you notice numbness in your feet or toes, it may be a sign that you need new shoes. Certainly, if your shoes are uncomfortable, stop wearing them and buy a new pair.

The Way Your Feet Look

You should not rely solely on how your feet feel to tell you if it is time to get new shoes. As you get older you may lose some of the feeling in your feet. You could be developing sores or calluses on your feet but not be aware of them if they are not painful. Check your feet daily to see if you have any new calluses or pressure areas. Usually callus or pressure areas mean your shoes are not fitting correctly. See Chapter 11 for further information on calluses and how to treat them.

The Condition of Your Old Shoes

You also should inspect your shoes to see if they need to be replaced. Make sure the soles are not slippery or excessively worn. It is important to replace your shoes if they are excessively worn since this will affect the way you walk. New aches and pains in your ankles, knees, and lower back may be related to the condition of your shoes.

Shopping for New Shoes

There are several things to keep in mind when shopping for new shoes.

1. Shop for shoes in the afternoon. Most people develop some swelling in their feet over the course of a day. If you try on new shoes in the afternoon, your feet usually will have swollen as much as they are likely to. By shopping in the afternoon, there is less chance of purchasing shoes that later will be too tight.

2. Purchase shoes that are the correct size. Make sure both shoes are wide enough and long enough for your feet when you are standing. Pay special attention to the fit across the ball of your foot because this segment widens as you get older. New shoes should be comfortable when you first try them on. It is not a good idea to buy shoes that need to be "broken in."

3. Look for padding inside the shoes. Always buy shoes with soft tops and shock absorbing foam insoles.

4. Pay attention to the kind of sole on the shoes. Make sure the sole of the shoe is not excessively slick and slippery. If possible, look for shoes with crepe soles because these best absorb the shock each time you take a step.

5. Avoid shoes with heels that are too high. A heel height of 1/2 inch usually is ideal.

6. If you do a lot of walking, it is a good idea to get athletic walking shoes. This type of shoe provides excellent foot support and extra cushioning in the soles.

7. If you have the choice, it is best to have a certified shoe fitter help you try on new shoes. These shoe fitters have specialized training in fitting shoes. Check shoe stores in your area to see which ones have certified shoe fitters.

Walking Barefoot

Never go barefoot! As you age, your skin becomes thinner and your circulation is not as good. Keeping your feet protected by wearing shoes is important for all older

people, but it is especially important for people with diabetes and circulation problems. Wear shoes during the day
and keep a pair of well-fitting slippers next to your bed to
put on if you have to get up in the middle of the night.

Wearing Socks

Socks alone are not a substitute for shoes or slippers.
They are almost always slippery and can easily contribute
to your falling. In addition, socks do not provide protection for your feet.

Avoid tight socks, panty hose, or garters that can cut off
your circulation. Unless your physician has prescribed the
use of compression socks to control swelling, your socks
should not feel constricting. Like shoes, socks should be
comfortable when you first put them on. They should not
bunch up at your toes or be tight around your ankles or
calves. Wearing clean, dry socks each day allows your feet
to "breathe" and will help reduce sweating.

Having Several Pairs of Shoes

Having several pairs of shoes that fit well is a good idea.
Alternating the shoes you wear can help prevent the formation of calluses. Each pair of shoes will have a slightly
different fit, therefore you will not have any one constant
pressure area from your shoes.

Special Shoes

Especially if you have problems with your feet, matching the shape of your foot needs to be the primary criteria when purchasing shoes. If you have had many foot problems in the past, you may need to have your shoes fit by a specialist called a pedorthist. Before seeing a pedorthist, however, you will need to see a physician or podiatrist to obtain a prescription for shoe adaptations.

Some shoe stores have trained pedorthists to help people with problem feet. Check in the yellow pages to see which shoe stores have pedorthists on staff. For a listing of pedorthists you can telephone the Prescription Footwear Association at 1-800-673-8447.

Summary

Well-fitting, comfortable footwear is a cornerstone to maintaining your mobility. Appropriate shoes serve several purposes. They protect your feet from injury, help relieve any discomfort you may have while walking, and aid in preventing calluses, sores, and toe deformities. Although having adequate shoes is the first step, making certain that you wear your footwear at all times when up and about is the second step. Wearing good, sturdy, comfortable shoes will help keep you mobile, active, and pain-free.

Chapter 13

Assistive Devices to Enhance Mobility

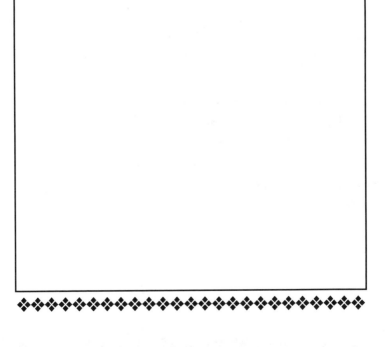

People have been using canes and crutches for centuries. Today there are many types of ambulation aids or assistive devices to choose from. There are various types of canes and crutches, plus two-, three-, and four-wheeled walkers and electric wheelchairs and scooters. Depending on your particular problem with mobility, one aid may be much more appropriate for you than another. Each type of assistive device is listed separately followed by a discussion of the benefits of that particular aid. Tips on the most effective way to use each device are also included.

Why Use an Ambulation Device?

There are six main reasons to use an assistive device:

1. Weakness. Many factors can cause a lack of strength, but whatever the cause, an assistive device often is helpful to compensate for muscle weakness.

2. Limited endurance. Using an assistive device often can allow you to walk greater distances. Frequently, you can be much more mobile with an ambulation aid than you would be without one.

3. Problems with balance. One of the main reasons many older people use an assistive device is to increase their stability. Using a walking device often improves balance.

4. Limited weight bearing. Often after a fracture, or following any type of leg surgery, you need to limit the amount of weight you put on that leg. Many assistive devices help you limit weight bearing. They allow you to shift some of the weight off of your leg and onto the assistive device.

5. Pain. Assistive devices can help if you have pain when you bear weight on one leg or the other. For example, if you have hip arthritis, using a cane can decrease the amount of hip pain you feel when you walk.

6. Fear of falling. After falling once, many people fear falling again. Using something to help you walk can allow you to remain mobile while decreasing your apprehension of falling again.

Often several of these reasons come into play for any one person. You may have pain in your knee from osteoarthritis and also have some problems with balance. Or you may need to limit the amount of weight you put on one leg following hip surgery and, at the same time, have muscle weakness. You also may have a fear of falling because you feel somewhat unsure of yourself after being in the hospital and outside your own environment for a period of time.

Types of Assistive Devices

There are very few hard and fast rules on what type of assistive device to use for any specific mobility problem. Therefore, if you or your doctor think you might benefit from an assistive device, you should be evaluated by a physical therapist to determine the best device for you.

Canes

For most people a cane is the least restrictive and easiest ambulation aid to use. With one exception, a cane can be used to help any of the problems listed at the start of this chapter. The one exception is if you need to severely limit the amount of weight you put on your leg. Only about 25% of your body weight can be transferred onto a cane, even if you lean very heavily on it as you walk. If you are recovering from orthopedic surgery, such as a hip replacement, and have been instructed to bear no more than 50% of your weight on your new hip, a cane would not work for you.

Tips on Using a Cane

Use a Cane on the Correct Side

You want to hold the cane on the side opposite of the leg that is causing you problems. If difficulty with balance, rather than weakness or pain, is the main reason you are using the cane, use the cane in the hand that feels most natural to you.

Make Sure Your Cane Is the Correct Height

When you are standing erect with your arm relaxed at your side, the handle of the cane should come to your wrist. Metal canes usually have a locking button for height adjustment. Wooden canes can be cut to the correct height by simply sawing off the bottom of the cane as needed.

How to Use a Cane

Begin by placing the cane in the hand opposite your sore leg. Next move the cane at the same time as your sore leg, so that as you step forward with your involved leg you also advance the cane forward. The cane gets moved ahead one step length, the same distance as you advance your leg. As you step onto your sore leg shift some of your weight onto the cane (see the illustration below). Just as when you walk without a cane, take steps of equal length with each foot as you use the cane. Keep the cane close to your side so you can easily rely on it to help you keep your balance.

Walking with Two Canes

If both legs are weak or painful, or if you feel more secure having something in both hands to steady yourself

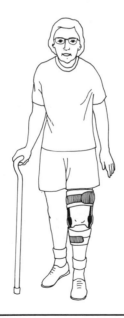

Walking with a cane.

with, you may benefit from using two canes. The same guidelines for using one cane apply when using two canes. Move the opposite cane and leg at the same time, just as your arms would naturally swing as you walk.

Going Up and Down Stairs

Certainly if there is a railing on stairs, use it! If there are two railings all the better. You can hook the end of your cane over your arm and hold onto both of the railings. If the stairway is wide and you are able to reach only one railing, hold onto the one that is on your strong side. When you start your climb up the stairs, firmly grasp the railing on your stronger side and transfer your cane to the opposite hand. Instead of the cane being on your stronger side as it is when you are walking, now it is on your weaker side, but you have the security and stability of a railing on your strong side.

Keeping the cane on the same step as your involved leg, step up onto the higher step with your strong leg, using the banister to help raise yourself up. Then advance your involved leg, along with the cane, up onto that step. Put both feet on each step, always putting your strong foot up onto the next step first (see illustration A on the next page). Continue this sequence until you reach the top of the stairs. Then transfer your cane back to your strong side where you use it for walking.

When going down stairs, you again want the railing on your stronger side if possible. Put the cane in your opposite hand. The cane gets moved to the step below first, so you can use it to lean on as you step down with your involved leg first, and then with your stronger leg. Your weak leg goes down the step first, followed by your stronger leg. As you lower yourself down to the step, your weight is supported by the leg remaining on the higher step, your stronger leg (see illustration B below).

If there is only one banister and it is on your weak side as you are descending the steps, it may be easiest for you to go down the stairs backwards. Standing with your back to the stairs, the railing is now on your stronger side. Some people use a backward descent regardless of the side of the railing because they feel safer using this method. The same principle applies for descending the steps. Put your

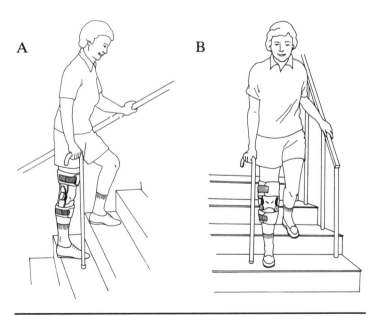

Negotiating stairs: A. Going up stairs. B. Going down stairs.

weaker leg down first, then lower your stronger leg. Keep the cane on the higher step because it is difficult to reach behind you to place it on the step below you.

Quad Canes

Four-legged canes, also called quad canes, come in two basic varieties: wide- and narrow-based. Depending on how much stability you need from a cane, either a wide or narrow type may be the best for you. Both offer significantly more stability than a single point cane does (see the illustration below). The technique for using a four-legged cane is basically the same as for using a single point cane; however, be certain that all four legs are firmly on the floor *before* you shift your weight onto the cane.

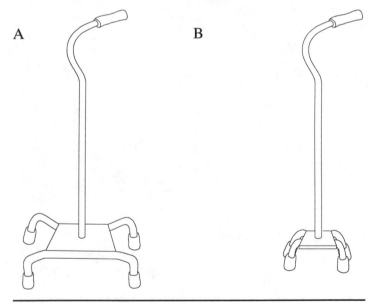

Quad canes. A. Wide based. B. Narrow based.

Crutches

Of all types of crutches, those that fit up under the arms are the most commonly used. These are the crutches we all are familiar with. Other types, such as Loftstrand and platform crutches, are less well known, but are very helpful in certain circumstances. Your physical therapist or physician can determine the best type of crutches for your particular needs.

Tips on Using Crutches

When you receive your crutches, you will be instructed in how to walk with them. There are several different ways to use crutches effectively, depending on how much weight you need to keep off each leg. If you are not sure of the gait pattern you were taught, check with your therapist or physician so they can review the particular gait pattern that is appropriate for you.

The tip to remember, no matter which type of crutches you have or what type of gait pattern you are using, is to stand as straight as possible with your crutches. You do not want to develop poor posture as a result of leaning too far forward while using your crutches.

Also, do not position yourself so your feet and crutches are all in a line. It is very easy to lose your balance and fall backwards if your crutches are positioned in the same line as your feet. When you are standing still, your crutches should be positioned slightly in front of your feet. By having your crutches slightly ahead of your feet, your base of support is larger and you are less likely to fall.

Walkers

There are several different types of walkers. Some come with wheels and some without; some with three wheels and some with four wheels and a seat. Each model has advantages and disadvantages, and no one style is always best for any single problem with mobility. A well-equipped physical therapy department will have a number of different walkers available for you to try. The physical therapist can help you determine which walker serves you best.

As with crutches, a variety of different gait patterns can be used with walkers. Your therapist or physician will need to instruct you in the proper way for you to effectively use your walker.

Almost all types of walkers can be folded to fit into a car. If you are going to be taking your walker outside your home, you will want one that is easy to fold and transport. Various types of baskets can be attached to walkers to allow you to carry items.

Four-Legged Walker

This is the type of walker people are most familiar with. Because there are no wheels, the walker must be picked up and advanced forward with each step, which makes walking slow. However this type of walker offers a lot of stability and can be used when all of your weight needs to be kept off one leg.

Walkers With Wheels

The advantage of having wheels on a walker is that it can be simply pushed along in front of you (see the illustration on page 217). As a result, it takes less work to use the walker, and walking is faster. A disadvantage is that you may find a wheeled walker too unsteady and may feel more stable using a walker without wheels.

Two-Wheeled Walkers

Most four-legged walkers can be modified by having wheels attached to the front two legs. A disadvantage of this type of walker is that the wheels move only in a single direction; they do not pivot (see illustration A on page 217).

However, there is a new type of walker which has two pivoting wheels on the front legs. Because the two front wheels pivot, this walker is quite maneuverable, and many people find it easy to use. For some people, however, it offers less stability than the two-wheeled nonpivoting walker.

Delta (Three-Wheeled) Walker. A delta is a new type of walker that has three wheels attached to a tripod style frame. The front wheel pivots in all directions which makes the walker very maneuverable and easy to use (see illustration B page 217). Because of its triangular frame, it fits more easily into small spaces than the traditional rectangular-style walker. Depending on the style of delta walker, it will have either hand brakes or brakes that lock the wheels when weight is applied downward on the handles. If a problem with balance is the primary reason you need to use an assistive device, a delta may be the best walker for you.

Four-Wheeled Walkers

A variety of companies now manufacture a walker with four wheels. Many of these walkers have seats which allow you to sit and rest as needed if you are walking longer distances (see illustration C on the next page). These walkers are more stable than delta walkers but have the disadvantage of being heavier and more difficult to maneuver in small spaces.

Other Aids to Maintaining Your Mobility

Even if you cannot walk, or cannot walk enough to be as active as you would like, there are aids that can help you maintain your mobility. These include various types of wheelchairs and scooters. You will need guidance from your physician or therapist to help you decide if using a wheelchair or scooter would be helpful.

There are many different sizes, styles, and features on wheelchairs and scooters. A therapist or trained salesperson can help you choose the model of wheelchair or scooter that is appropriate for you.

Companion Chair

This is a unique type of wheeled chair that has small tires in place of the large rear tires that wheelchairs have (see the illustration page 218). The advantage of having small wheels is that the chair is very lightweight and easy to transport. The back of the chair folds down which adds to the ease of getting it in and out of a car. A companion

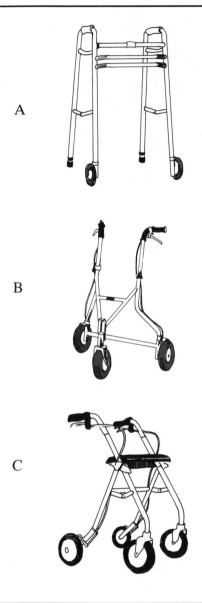

Wheeled walkers: A. Two-wheeled pivoting. B. Delta (three-wheeled). C. Four-wheeled.

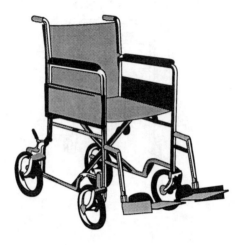

Companion wheelchair.

chair can be an ideal wheeled chair to keep in the trunk of a car and use on outings when a lot of walking is required.

A disadvantage of the back tires being small is that you cannot reach them to use your hands to propel this type of chair. It can be propelled using your feet, but most people find a companion chair works best by having someone else push it.

Manual Wheelchairs

All manual wheelchairs have essentially the same basic design but come in a variety of different sizes. There are subtle differences between brands and styles of wheelchairs that can make a big difference in using them. If you will be using a wheelchair for an extended period, it would be wise to have a therapist or trained salesperson evaluate you to determine the best size and model for you. This way you will have a wheelchair that fits your build and has the features you need.

You may prefer to rent rather than buy a wheelchair. Particularly if you think you are only going to be using the wheelchair for a couple months, renting may be cheaper than buying. If you think you are going to be using the wheelchair for a long time, then buying it probably makes more sense financially. Whether you buy or rent, however, you should get a wheelchair that is the correct size and has the features that are appropriate for you.

Things to Consider When Renting or Buying a Wheelchair

Size. The first factor to consider when getting a wheelchair is what the proper size is for you. Standard size wheelchairs have a seat depth and width of 18 inches. A narrow wheelchair has a depth of 18 inches but a width of only 16 inches. Although not appropriate for large adults, a narrow wheelchair fits a small adult quite well.

Wheelchair Back. The backs of wheelchairs come in different heights. A tall-backed chair can give your back and neck extra support if you need it.

Armrest Height. Arm height is also variable. The armrest should be positioned so that your forearm sits comfortably on it. Especially if you are short, you may benefit from a lower height armrest so your shoulders are not hunched up when your elbows are on the armrest.

Desk Armrests. One of the features on wheelchairs that you may find helpful is a "desk armrest." This type of armrest is cut down in the front so the wheelchair can fit up close to a desk or table.

Seat Length. Seat length is another important component to consider. If you have long legs you may need extra length in the seat to be comfortable. Your thighs should be securely supported by the seat of the wheelchair.

Wheelchair Cushions. If you are going to be sitting in a wheelchair for any period of time, you will need some type of padding on the seat to be comfortable. When you first purchase or rent a wheelchair, get a cushion at the same time. A foam cushion usually is adequate as long as you are not sitting in the wheelchair all the time.

If you sit in your wheelchair for long periods of time, you will want a special type of cushion that distributes your weight more evenly. Gel or air-filled cushions and high density foam are examples of cushions that provide extra comfort and support.

Basic foam cushions are the least expensive. High quality cushions cost many times more. Medical supply stores carry various types of cushions. A therapist or knowledgeable salesperson can advise you on what type of cushion would be most appropriate for you.

Tires. Other features to consider in a wheelchair are the types of tires. Some tires are air-filled whereas others are solid so that they do not go flat. Solid tires are easier to propel on smooth hard surfaces such as wood and vinyl floors. One drawback to solid tires is that they generally don't provide as smooth a ride outdoors or on uneven surfaces as air-filled tires.

Safety Precautions. Whatever wheelchair you may use, you should be sure the brakes work well and that the chair is always locked securely before you get in or out of it. It is all too easy for a wheelchair to roll away from you if the wheels are not firmly locked.

Electric Wheelchairs

If you are unable to walk or can only take a few steps and cannot propel a manual wheelchair, an electric wheelchair may be what you need to maintain your mobility. Electric wheelchairs are very expensive, but in some cases may be partially paid for by Medicare or by your health insurance.

Like manual wheelchairs, electric wheelchairs are available in a wide variety of sizes, features, and options. A therapist can help you decide what chair is best for you. As with a manual wheelchair, you will need a comfortable cushion to sit on. Your therapist also can advise you on the best type of cushion.

Scooters

A scooter is a three-wheeled, battery powered cart that can be ideal for someone who cannot walk long distances (see the illustration on the next page). Many models are rear wheel driven and provide enough power to easily

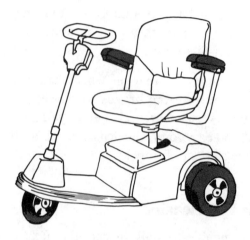

Scooter.

get around outdoors and on uneven surfaces. Smaller models of scooters have front wheel drives and are designed primarily for indoor use.

All models are costly but some brands are significantly less expensive than others. Front wheel drives generally are cheaper than rear wheel drives. As with electric wheelchairs, in some cases Medicare or health insurance may cover some of the cost.

Buying a scooter is somewhat similar to deciding on what make and model of car to buy. Features can be quite different and one model is not inherently better than another. It depends on which scooter fits you best and has the options you need. Things like seat height adjustment, drive mechanisms, speed variation, and armrests are several of the factors to consider when purchasing a scooter.

Most scooters have a cushion built into the seat, similar to a car seat. Again, you need to find a seat that is comfortable for you. If you'd like, an additional cushion usually can be placed over the seat cushion to improve comfort.

A trained salesperson can show you different types of scooters and explain the options available. Be sure to test drive any scooter that you are considering. Ideally, you should try the scooter out in your own home. You want to be certain you will be able to easily charge the battery and that you will be able to store it in an accessible place. The most important thing is to get a scooter that works well in the environment where you will be using it.

Summary

People are often hesitant to use an ambulation aid, be it a simple cane or a four-wheeled walker. They are concerned that they will come to depend too much on the device and lose the ability to walk without it. However, only rarely does this happen. If using an ambulation aid allows you to increase your mobility, then by all means take advantage of it!

The ultimate goal is to maintain or improve your mobility. Use a three-wheeled walker, or a cane, or whatever type of device suits your needs to allow you to walk. Don't let the fear of what others may think interfere with your independence! By using an assistive device you may be able to walk farther, and more safely, than you could without the aid. People will pay very little attention to whatever type of ambulation aid you are using. Rather, they will be happy to see you continue to walk!

Chapter 14

Falls and Home Safety

❖❖❖❖❖❖❖❖❖❖❖❖❖❖❖❖❖❖❖❖❖❖❖❖❖❖❖❖❖❖❖❖❖❖❖

You are bound to experience many falls during your lifetime. Think of how often you fell as a toddler when you were first learning to walk, or how as a school-age child, you fell when you were running, jumping, or playing outside. But as you age, falling becomes something to be more and more cautious of and to prevent as much as possible.

What Causes Falls?

Studies that asked people why they fell show that people often aren't certain of the cause of their falls. Answers included: "I just fell," "I must have tripped," "My legs gave way," or "I guess I lost my balance."

As you can imagine, a multitude of factors can contribute to someone falling. Most falls are not the result of only one cause; usually several factors play a role. For instance, when someone slips in the kitchen, a wet floor may apparently have been the cause. But at the same time maybe the person was wearing slippers with slick soles or socks but no shoes. Perhaps the person also was in a hurry to answer the telephone and was lightheaded from getting up too quickly out of the chair. As you can see, really this fall was related to several factors. The slippery floor was only one reason the person fell.

Not paying attention and attempting risky or unsafe maneuvers are common contributors to falls. You may fall trying to carry two bags of groceries up a flight of stairs. Or you may not notice ice on the sidewalk or water on the kitchen floor. Research has shown that in most cases people who have fallen think that their falls could have been prevented if they had paid more attention or been more careful when they were walking.

Certainly many hazards in a person's surroundings also can contribute to falls. Most falls occur in the home and tripping over objects on the floor is a very common problem. Throw rugs, clutter on the floor, and telephone cords strung across the room can easily be hazards even for young people in the best of health. Think how much more hazardous these things can be for an older person whose eyesight and balance are not quite as good!

Who is Likely to Fall?

Some of the major risk factors that predispose people to falling are listed below. The likelihood of falling depends on how many of these risk factors you have.

1. Your overall health. If you are in poor health and physical condition, you are more likely to fall than if your health is good. When your health is poor, your reaction time is slower, your muscles are weaker, and you fatigue more easily.

2. Muscle weakness. Muscle weakness, especially weakness of the leg muscles, can make you much more susceptible to falling. Chapter 3 gives exercises which may help you to strengthen your muscles and decrease your risk for falls.

3. Vision impairment. If you cannot see well, you will be more likely to stumble or trip over objects. If you have problems with depth perception, you may find it more difficult to step off curbs or go up and down stairs. If you have trouble with glare, high gloss floors and wet surfaces can be much more hazardous for you. Chapter 10 discusses some common conditions that can affect your eyesight and increase your risk for falls.

4. Balance problems. If you have trouble with your balance, no matter what the cause, your risk of falling is increased. Chapter 1 explains what makes up your sense of balance, and Chapters 7 and 10 discuss various diseases that can lead to problems with balance.

5. Medications. Some medications can make you weak or lightheaded, others can slow your reaction time or affect your coordination. Some medications that cause dizziness or lightheadedness are discussed in Chapter 7. Chapter 10 gives additional information about medications that can affect your mobility and predispose you to falling.

What Happens When Older People Fall?

Injuries Related to Falling

Fortunately, most falls do not cause serious injury. Roughly 5% of falls result in a broken bone. For younger adults the most common bone broken in a fall is the wrist; for older people hip fractures are more common.

Injuries such as sprains, cuts, and bruises frequently occur as a result of falling. At times these injuries can be serious enough to require medical care. A severe bump on the head from a fall can be life-threatening and always needs to be evaluated to be certain there is not bleeding around the brain. Also, if you lose consciousness after a fall you should be seen by a physician to determine the extent of the injury.

Fear Of Falling

Almost half of all people who fall develop a fear of falling. One quarter of those who fall limit their activities because they are afraid of falling again. A certain amount of fear of falling and using common sense to avoid a fall is healthy. However, an excessive fear of falling can cause you to restrict your mobility more than is reasonable. Cutting back on walking and other activities can lead to a decrease in strength and endurance. Your cardiac system gets deconditioned and your mood can become depressed. Therefore, although you need to be cautious to avoid a fall, it is very important to stay as active and mobile as you can.

Nursing Homes

Usually a single fall does not lead to a nursing home admission. However, if you fall repeatedly, it may be very difficult for you to continue to live independently. The decision to move to a nursing home is a very difficult one. Although a nursing home may be a safer environment, it can also restrict your mobility and limit your independence. Before you consider moving to a nursing home because you are falling, see your physician to find out why you are falling and what you can do to prevent falls.

If you have received a medical evaluation to determine the cause of your falls, and followed your doctor's advice regarding treatment, but continue to fall, you and your family may need to consider the option of moving to a nursing home. It is important to remember, however, that it should never be the first option that you consider after a fall. *Coping with Loss of Independence*, another book in the Coping with Aging Series, contains detailed information on nursing homes.

What To Do If You Fall

Getting Up

Falling can be a frightening experience, but it is important to remain as calm as possible after you fall. Keep your wits about you and assess the situation. If you do not appear to be injured, slowly and cautiously get up if you can.

Many times even when people are not injured from falling they are not able to get up easily. It may help you to scoot or crawl to a piece of furniture or something in the environment that you can use to help pull yourself up.

Getting Help If You Can't Get Up

Calling out for help will often attract someone's attention. If no one is around to help you and you can reach a telephone, call a neighbor or family member. It may be beneficial to have a portable telephone that you keep near you. It also is a good idea to keep a list of neighbors' telephone numbers on the telephone because you may not be able to remember the telephone numbers when you are in a crisis.

If no neighbor or family member is available to help you get up, and you are able to reach the telephone, you can call the police. If you are not hurt there is no need for an ambulance, but the services of a police officer, or some-one they may send, can be used to help lift you up.

If you have problems with your mobility, it is a good idea to have someone check on you at least once, and prefer-ably more often, every day. You do not want to be caught in a situation where you fall and lie on the floor for a long time waiting for help.

Lifeline

If you have fallen before, or if you have several risk fac-tors for falling, a Lifeline service may be one of the best investments you can make. This service provides you with a small device which you wear around your neck or wrist. Lifeline is similar to a telephone service.If you fall, you push a button on the device and a person whom you have designated ahead of time as your contact is called automatically. This person receives your call and then checks up on you to make sure you are all right. If your contact doesn't answer the telephone your call automati-cally is transferred to a central number where someone is available at all times to get help for you.

Lifeline is a local service, and in each locale it may be run slightly differently. Usually you pay a monthly fee for the service. Although you may think the cost high and the service unnecessary, you should seriously consider it if your mobility is impaired. Especially if you live alone, Lifeline may be the key to staying independent! You can contact a local hospital or senior citizen's group to find out more about the program in your area.

Evaluating a Fall

Evaluate a fall by thinking of all the circumstances and factors that could have played a role in the accident. How much did the environment contribute to your falling? What factors inherent to you played a part? What you want to do is to learn from your fall, so similar falls can be avoided in the future. Maybe you need to be extra cautious when walking on uneven surfaces. Possibly you need to use a cane when you are outside, especially at night or when there is poor light. Perhaps you could benefit from pacing your activities so fatigue doesn't increase your chances of losing your balance and falling.

The more things you can do to prevent falling, the less likely you will be to fall. As mentioned earlier, most falls have more than one contributing factor. Try to think of as many factors and as many interventions as possible so that you can prevent similar falls from occurring.

Notifying Your Doctor

Certainly if you are injured in a fall, even if you think the injury is minor, you should call your doctor. Also, if you had any feelings of faintness or lightheadedness, or felt ill prior to or right after a fall, your doctor will want to know about it sooner rather than later.

Falls are not a normal part of growing older. Instead, they often are a signal that you have some underlying condition or problem that should be treated. Be sure to tell your doctor if you have fallen recently.

Maintaining Independence After a Fall

There are many things you can do to ensure you maintain your independence after a fall. You may need to change some of your habits, such as no longer shopping in a mall that requires you to walk long distances if you now have muscle soreness. Instead, shop at only one store at a time or find a store that can deliver to you. You may want to take a shower versus a tub bath if you have difficulty getting in and out of the bathtub because of joint stiffness after a fall. You may need to rely on other people for help with things like laundry, yard work, and housekeeping. Your physician or local senior citizen organization can give you information on obtaining chore services or other support so that you can remain as independent as possible.

If fear of falling is limiting your confidence when going out, using an assistive device or having someone with you can be the answer to maintaining your independence. Following an exercise program also can help you regain your confidence after a fall. Chapters 3 and 5 describe a number of exercises which can increase your strength and flexibility after a fall. The key is to regain your mobility and resume your normal activities as quickly as possible.

What You Can Do to Prevent Falls

In the case of falls, an ounce of prevention is worth a pound of cure. If you don't fall, you don't have to be concerned about losing your mobility because of an injury resulting from falling. However, although you want to be reasonably cautious to prevent a fall, you don't want to stop being active. What you want to do is avoid taking unnecessary chances with dangerous behaviors and unsafe environments.

Walk Safely

Try to keep your steps even and consistent so your walking pattern is smooth and flowing. Everyone's gait pattern is different. No matter what your natural walking pattern, you can strive to maintain a smooth, even walking sequence. If you have an assistive device such as a cane or walker, and it helps you to walk safely, be sure to use it. Chapter 13 discusses assistive devices that are available to help people maintain their mobility and reduce their risk of falling.

Transfer Safely

Transfers are movements made to get from one position to another that do not involve walking. For example, getting into bed from sitting on a bedside chair and getting in and out of a car are transfer movements.

Going From Standing to Sitting

Being aware of where your body is, relative to where you want to get to, is especially important when doing any stand-to-sit transfer. Be certain that you have a firm hold on the piece of furniture or place you are moving toward. For example, if you are getting into a car, securely grasp the door handle and reach back for the seat before you sit down. Many falls occur because people sit down before they are close enough to the seat or because a chair slides out from under them.

Going From Sitting to Standing

Use your hands to help push yourself up when going from a sitting to a standing position. This will make standing up less jerky. Also, scooting forward in a chair prior to standing will make getting up much easier. You want to get your center of gravity as far forward over your feet as possible.

Proper Chair Height. Ideally, the seat should be at the same level as the back of your knees. Sitting on chairs with the proper seat height improves your body mechanics as you go from sitting to standing. Everyone has experienced how much harder it is to get up from sitting in a low, soft cushioned sofa or chair compared to rising from a high, firm chair. If a chair at home is too low, you can add a firm foam cushion to the seat to make it the correct height.

Transferring in the Bathroom

Toilet Transfers. If you have problems transferring to and from the toilet, there are several things you can do. The height of a toilet seat can easily be raised by adding a raised toilet seat (see the illustration below). You also can purchase toilet rails to help with transferring. Medical supply stores carry a variety of styles of elevated toilet seats and toilet rails that you can choose from.

Tub and Shower Transfer. If you have problems getting in or out of the tub, place grab bars on the tub wall or in the shower. Grab bars placed around a shower or tub area are very helpful in preventing falls and increasing your mobility by giving you something to hold onto as you transfer. Also to prevent falls, be sure you have non-slip appliques on the bottom of the tub.

Tub Seats. You also may want to consider using a bathtub seat or bench. If sitting down in the tub to bathe or

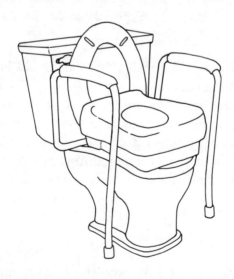

Toilet rails and elevated seat.

standing up to take a shower is difficult for you, sitting on a bench as you bathe or shower can be a big help. Some tub benches have back- and armrests which you may find useful. Most seats have height adjustments so they can be raised to a comfortable position for you. Because not all brands fit in all tubs or showers, you will need to make sure a particular seat will work in your home.

Preventing Falls Outside the Home

Besides the inside of your home, your environment includes other areas such as the yard outside your home, the car or taxi you use, and the stores where you shop. Do you always use the railing when boarding the bus or subway? When the sidewalk is slippery from rain or snow, do you move extra cautiously and avoid distractions such as talking when you need to concentrate on walking and keeping your balance? Are there benches or chairs to sit on if you become tired when shopping? Plan your shopping trips for a time when the stores are least busy so the congestion of a lot of people is not a hazard to falling.

Preventing Falls Inside the Home

Because most falls occur in the home, pay close attention to your home environment when thinking of reducing the risk of falls. Look objectively throughout your home and make any changes necessary to improve the safety of your environment.

If you are not sure how to evaluate your home for hazards, a physical or occupational therapist can help. A therapist can come to your home and check to see whether the stairs, rooms, and walkways are as safe as possible for you. Your doctor can arrange a home safety evaluation from a professional. At times Medicare will pay for this service.

Tips for Improving Home Safety

Improving home safety does not have to be an expensive or time-consuming task. Below are a number of very simple things you can do to help make your home as safe as possible.

Exterior

1. Provide good lighting for the outdoor area. Pay special attention to the lighting around sidewalks and entrances because these are heavily used areas.

2. Check the sidewalks and walkways for large cracks that might make walking unsafe. Notify your local Public Works Department if you find public sidewalks that are hazardous.

3. Check lawns and gardens for holes and uneven surfaces. Have holes filled in if you can, and be aware of uneven areas so you don't inadvertently trip.

Home Interior

1. Be sure you have good lighting throughout your home. Especially if you have problems with your balance, good lighting can help reduce your risk of falling.

2. Make sure light switches are easy to reach in all rooms. This is especially true in the bedroom, where a lamp should be easily reachable from the bed. Also be sure you have night lights in hallways and bathrooms.

3. Keep clutter off the floor and steps. Many falls are due to tripping over objects. Keeping the floors clear of objects you could trip over may be the best way to reduce falls.

4. Remove throw rugs or securely tape them down. Wide double-sided tape, which you can purchase in hardware stores, works well. Also make sure carpet edges are fastened down securely and not loose or fraying.

5. Keep telephone cords out of the way of traffic. All wires and cords should be close to the wall where you cannot trip over them.

6. If you have difficulty crossing door thresholds, place a small grab rail by the doorway to give you extra support (see the illustration on the next page).

7. Avoid using high gloss wax on floors because glare can obscure your vision and the slick wax can make walking treacherous.

Stairs

Ten percent or more of all falls within the home occur on stairs. The bottom step usually gives the most trouble, and falls occur more frequently going down stairs rather than up.

1. Make sure there are sturdy handrails on all stairs. Ideally, you want handrails on both sides of a flight of stairs.

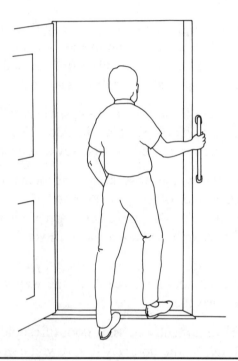

Grab rail by doorway.

2. Be sure you have light switches at the top and bottom of the steps. Good illumination is essential for preventing falls.

3. Check the carpeting on the stairs to make sure it is not too plush. Ideally the carpeting should be very low pile without a lot of padding because a firm surface helps improve foot stability.

4. Patterned carpet makes it harder to tell where the edge of the step is. If you have trouble seeing where each stair ends, place a strip of colored tape along the edge of each step.

Kitchen

1. If you have trouble reaching high cupboards, place frequently used kitchen items at about shoulder height. If bending and stooping are hard for you, arrange the most frequently used items high enough so you do not have to bend over to reach them.

2. Check your kitchen floor to make sure it is not slippery. And, of course, remember to wipe up all spills as soon as they occur. If you have mats on the kitchen floor, be certain they are nonskid.

Summary

The best way to treat the problem of falling is to prevent falls from occurring in the first place. Improving safety in your environment and reducing as many risk factors as possible are two very important ways to prevent falls. Keeping safety a priority will decrease your risk of falling and allow you to maintain your mobility as much as possible.

Appendix

Sources for
Additional Information

General Information

American Association of Retired Persons
601 E Street NW
Washington, DC 20049
800-424-3410

Resources on many issues related to older persons, including free booklets on improving mobility, fitness and exercise for older adults, and home safety.

Consumer Information Catalog
P.O. Box 100
Pueblo, CO 81009
713-948-3334

Has many free or low-cost federal publications on health and exercise, specific medical problems, and Medicare benefits.

National Health Information Center
P.O. Box 1133
Washington, DC 20012-1133
800-336-4797

Provides referrals to over 1,000 health organizations and distributes publications containing resource and referral information, some specifically targeted for older adults.

National Institute on Aging
Information Center
P.O. Box 8057
Gaithersburg, MD 20893-8057
800-222-2225

Puts out a free fact sheet "AGE PAGE Preventing Falls and Fractures" for older adults. Also offers other free publications on health and aging.

Arthritis (Chapter 8)

Arthritis Foundation
1314 Spring Street NW
Atlanta, GA 30309
800-283-7800

Has educational materials about arthritis and provides information about Arthritis Foundation chapters around the country.

Osteoporosis (Chapter 9)

National Osteoporosis Foundation
1150 17th Street NW, Suite 500
Washington, DC 20037
800-223-9994

Has educational materials on osteoporosis including a free 22-page brochure "Stand Up to Osteoporosis."

Conditions Affecting Mobility (Chapter 10)

Alzheimer's Disease and Related Disorders Association
919 N Michigan Ave
Chicago, IL 60611
800-621-0379

Offers a free information packet on Alzheimer's disease and provides referrals to local support groups and chapters.

American Association for the Visually Handicapped
22 West 21st Street
New York, NY 10010
212-889-3141

Has free large print newsletters and a catalog on visual aids. Also provides referrals to resources in your area.

American Diabetes Association
1660 Duke Street
Alexandria, VA 22314
800-232-3472

Provides educational information and a newsletter related to diabetes.

American Heart Association
7272 Greenville Avenue
Dallas, TX 75231
800-242-1793

Provides information on cardiac conditions and preventative measures you can take to limit heart disease.

American Lung Association
1740 Broadway
New York, NY 10019
800-586-4872

Offers brochures on many topics related to lung diseases and health issues concerning breathing. Also provides information regarding associations in your area.

American Parkinson Disease Association
60 Bay Street, Suite 401
Staten Island, NY 10301
800-223-2732

Offers information about local chapters and support groups; also publishes a booklet "Be Active: A Suggested Exercise Program for People with Parkinson's Disease."

National Stroke Association
8480 E. Orchard Road, Suite 1000
Englewood, CO 80111-5015
800-7870-6537

Provides information for stroke survivors and their families on treatment, risk factors and adaptive aids.

Feet and Footwear (Chapters 11 and 12)

Prescription Footwear Association
9861 Broken Land Parkway, Suite 255
Columbia, MD 21046
800-673-8447

Write or call with your shoe length and width for a listing of stores in your area that carry your size. Free publication on 10 points of proper shoe fit. Also has referrals to certified pedorthists in your area.

Home Safety and Adaptive Equipment (Chapter 14)

National Safety Council
P.O. Box 558
Itasca, IL 60143-0558
800-621-7619

Publishes a free home safety checklist and other publications including "Preventing Falls."

U.S. Consumer Product Safety Commission
Washington, D.C. 20207
Attention: Publications Requests
301-504-0580

Offers a free home safety checklist for older consumers.

Enrichments
P.O. Box 471, Dept C58
Western Springs, IL 60558-9900
800-323-5547

Has a free catalog of affordable items to improve home safety and mobility.

Sears Health Care
P.O. Box 19009
Provo, UT 84605
800-326-1750.

Call for a free catalog of adaptive equipment and home health aids sold by Sears.

Index